By Mila Grace

Yoga After 60:

Embracing Health and Flexibility Through Holistic Practices

7-Day Yoga Challenge:

Day-by-Day Guidance for a Transformative Journey

Contents

Chapter I
Introduction to Yoga for Seniors and Beginners

Welcome to the beginning of a transformative journey—a path that intertwines the wisdom of your years with the timeless teachings of yoga. This journey is more than merely a physical endeavor; it is an invitation to explore the depth of your being, to enhance your quality of life, and to embrace the golden years with vigor, grace, and serenity.

Yoga, a practice with ancient roots, has flourished across cultures and epochs, offering its rich tapestry of benefits to all who seek its wisdom. For seniors, yoga presents a unique and powerful opportunity to nurture the body, calm the mind, and replenish the spirit. As we step into this practice, we recognize that yoga for seniors is not about perfection or performance; it's about meeting yourself where you are, honoring your journey, and embracing the art of possibility.

Embracing Your Journey with Yoga
The beauty of yoga lies in its adaptability and inclusiveness. Regardless of your physical condition, mobility level, or previous experience, yoga has a place for you. It's a practice that grows with you, offering gentle stretches for flexibility, postures for strength, and breathing exercises for deep relaxation. Each element of yoga is a step towards achieving a harmonious balance between body and mind, fostering physical and emotional well-being.

The Physical Benefits: A Gateway to Vitality
For many seniors, the physical benefits of yoga are the initial draw. Regular practice can significantly enhance flexibility, making daily activities more accessible and enjoyable. Strength-building poses work to fortify the muscles and bones, reducing the risk of falls and improving overall stability. Moreover, yoga's emphasis on balance can transform your physical poise, instilling confidence in every step.

But yoga's gifts extend far beyond flexibility and balance. It is a powerful ally in managing chronic conditions such as arthritis, hypertension, and diabetes. Through gentle movements and mindful breathing, yoga encourages a deeper connection with the body, enabling practitioners to navigate their health with greater awareness and care.

The Mental and Emotional Harmony: Beyond the Physical
Yoga's impact on mental and emotional well-being is profound. In a world that often feels hurried and chaotic, yoga offers a sanctuary of peace and presence. Practices like meditation and pranayama (breath control) are integral to yoga, guiding seniors toward a state of mindfulness that alleviates stress, anxiety, and depression. This mindful awareness enhances quality of life, promoting a sense of contentment, gratitude, and joy in everyday moments.

A Community of Support and Growth
Embarking on your yoga journey introduces you to a community of fellow travelers, each with their own stories and experiences. This sense of belonging can be profoundly enriching, offering support, motivation, and friendship. Together, you'll explore the realms of yoga, sharing

insights, challenges, and breakthroughs. The community you find in yoga can become a source of strength and encouragement, reminding you that you are not alone on this path.

Your Invitation

As you stand at the threshold of this journey, know that yoga is not just an activity—it's a way of living, a practice that enriches every facet of your being. It invites you to explore, grow, and discover a world of wellness that transcends age. Yoga for seniors is a celebration of life, an acknowledgment of your strength, and a testament to your resilience.

Welcome to yoga. Welcome to a journey of transformation, healing, and profound joy. Let us embrace this path with open hearts and curious minds as we explore the boundless possibilities that await.

The Importance of Yoga in Later Life

Embracing yoga in later life is not just physical exercise; it's a profound commitment to enhancing your overall well-being, vitality, and joy during the golden years. As we navigate the complexities of aging, yoga emerges as a beacon of hope, offering a path to improved health, increased flexibility, and more profound inner peace. This journey through yoga is not merely about bending and stretching; it's about discovering a more profound sense of self, embracing tranquility, and fostering a connection between mind, body, and spirit that flourishes with time.

The importance of yoga in later life cannot be overstated. It is a powerful antidote to the challenges that often accompany aging. Through gentle stretches and mindful breathing, yoga helps alleviate joint pain, enhance mobility, and reduce the risk of falls by improving balance and strength. But the benefits of yoga extend far beyond the physical. It is a source of mental and emotional rejuvenation, reducing stress, enhancing mood, and cultivating a sense of well-being that is invaluable at any age.

Our worlds sometimes feel smaller as we age, but yoga encourages a boundless exploration of our capabilities and potential. It invites seniors to redefine their limitations to find growth and possibilities within themselves that they might never have imagined. Yoga practices tailored for seniors are not about reaching the highest level of physical achievement but about honoring the body's needs, celebrating progress, and embracing each moment with gratitude and mindfulness.

Moreover, yoga fosters a sense of community and connection. Joining a class or practice group introduces seniors to like-minded individuals, forming bonds over shared experiences and mutual support. This sense of belonging can be profoundly impactful, breaking through the isolation that too often accompanies later life and knitting together the fabric of a community anchored in health, mindfulness, and mutual respect.

In embracing yoga, we find a practice and a philosophy of living that enriches our golden years. It teaches us to live with intention, breathe purposefully, and move through life's challenges with grace and resilience. Yoga is a testament to the enduring strength of the human spirit, a reminder that it is never too late to seek balance, strive for harmony, and pursue a life filled with peace, joy, and fulfillment.

Let yoga be your guide to a vibrant, fulfilling life in your later years. It promises a healthier body and a sanctuary for the soul, a place where every breath brings you closer to your essence; every pose strengthens your muscles and your resolve, and every practice is a step towards a more luminous, serene, and enriched life. Embrace this journey with open arms, and let the transformative power of yoga illuminate your path.

Debunking Myths About Yoga and Age

As a seasoned practitioner and advocate of yoga, I've encountered numerous misconceptions that can deter seniors from embracing this transformative practice. The myths surrounding yoga and age are pervasive, yet with understanding and insight, we can dispel these falsehoods and open the door to a world of wellness and vitality for individuals in their golden years. Here, we address and debunk the most common myths about yoga and age, illuminating the truth of yoga's accessibility and its profound benefits for seniors.

Myth 1: "Yoga is only for the young and flexible."
One of the most widespread myths is that yoga is exclusive to the young and inherently flexible. This couldn't be further from the truth. Yoga is a practice that welcomes all, regardless of age or flexibility level. It's not about performing complex poses perfectly but meeting your body where it is. For seniors, yoga offers numerous modifications and variations, ensuring that poses are accessible and beneficial. The essence of yoga lies in its adaptability, making it a perfect fit for seniors eager to enhance their flexibility, strength, and balance at any starting point.

Myth: "Yoga is not a good enough workout for older adults."
Many believe that yoga lacks the intensity older adults need for it to be considered a "real workout." This misconception overlooks the variety within yoga practices, ranging from gentle and restorative to more vigorous and challenging styles. Yoga for seniors can be tailored to provide cardiovascular benefits, strengthen muscles, and improve endurance, all while being mindful of safety and individual physical limitations. The intensity of a yoga session can be adjusted to match and challenge the practitioner's ability, making it a comprehensive workout that holistically addresses the body's needs.

Myth 3: "It's too late to start yoga if you're already a senior."
The belief that there's a "right" age to start yoga is a significant barrier for many seniors. However, yoga is a journey that knows no age limit. Starting yoga later in life can still yield tremendous benefits, including improved mobility, enhanced mental clarity, and reduced symptoms of chronic conditions. Yoga encourages a mindful awareness of the body and breath, fostering a sense of well-being that is invaluable at any stage of life. It's never too late to begin, and yoga offers a path to improved health and happiness tailored to the unique needs of older practitioners.

Myth 4: "Yoga is not safe for seniors with health issues."
Concerns about safety and health conditions often prevent seniors from exploring yoga. While it's essential to consult with a healthcare provider before beginning any new exercise regimen, yoga is widely recognized for its adaptability and the gentle approach it offers. Specialized yoga classes for seniors, including those with health issues like arthritis, osteoporosis, and heart conditions, are designed to provide safe, supportive environments where poses are modified to accommodate specific needs. Yoga instructors trained in working with seniors can

guide practitioners through sequences that enhance health without exacerbating existing conditions.

The Reality

The reality is that yoga is a gateway to improved physical, mental, and emotional health for seniors. It debunks myths with every gentle stretch, balanced pose, and mindful breath. It offers a holistic approach to wellness that respects the body's limitations while celebrating its capabilities. By embracing yoga, seniors can discover renewed vitality, strength, and joy in their golden years.

In debunking these myths, we invite seniors to explore the enriching world of yoga, a practice that supports a vibrant, healthy, and fulfilling life at any age. Let us shed these misconceptions and step into the empowering, inclusive embrace of yoga together.

How Yoga Benefits Seniors

With its holistic approach to well-being, yoga offers many benefits tailored to seniors' unique needs. This ancient practice goes beyond physical exercises, promoting mental clarity, emotional balance, and inner peace. As we delve into the specific ways yoga benefits seniors, it becomes clear why this practice is not just beneficial but essential for aging gracefully and healthily.

Physical Health Enhancements

Improved Flexibility and Mobility: Regular yoga practice gently stretches and tones the body, enhancing flexibility and mobility. This is particularly beneficial for seniors, as it can lead to improved posture, reduced stiffness, and decreased aches and pains associated with aging.

Increased Strength and Balance: Yoga poses (asanas) strengthen muscles and improve balance, which is crucial for seniors to maintain independence and reduce the risk of falls. Balancing exercises in yoga can also enhance coordination and proprioception, helping seniors feel more stable and confident in their movements.

Enhanced Joint Health: Yoga promotes joint health by improving circulation and flexibility, which can benefit seniors with arthritis or osteoporosis. Gentle movements encourage synovial fluid production, providing lubrication and aiding in easing joint pain.

Mental and Cognitive Benefits

Stress Reduction and Improved Mental Clarity: Yoga incorporates breathing exercises (pranayama) and meditation (dhyana), which help calm the mind, reduce stress, and enhance mental clarity. This can translate into better sleep patterns, reduced anxiety, and a more positive outlook for seniors.

Enhanced Cognitive Function: Regular yoga practice has been linked to improvements in cognitive function, including memory, attention, and concentration. This is particularly relevant for seniors, as maintaining mental health is critical to aging.

Emotional Balance: Yoga's meditative aspect encourages practitioners to focus on the present, fostering an attitude of mindfulness that can lead to more excellent emotional stability and a reduction in feelings of depression and loneliness.

Social and Spiritual Well-being

Community and Connection: Joining a yoga class gives seniors community and belonging. Connecting with others in a supportive environment reduces feelings of isolation. Yoga's emphasis on compassion and self-understanding can also enhance relationships with oneself and others.

Spiritual Growth: For many seniors, yoga provides a pathway to spiritual exploration and growth. It encourages a deeper connection with one's inner self, fostering a sense of peace, contentment, and fulfillment that transcends physical health.

Lifestyle Integration: Yoga offers a holistic approach to health that can extend beyond the mat. It encourages healthy eating habits, positive thinking, and a mindful approach to everyday activities. This integration into daily life can significantly improve the quality of life for seniors.

In essence, yoga offers seniors a comprehensive toolkit for navigating the challenges of aging. It provides a sustainable practice for maintaining physical health, supports mental and cognitive well-being, and fosters emotional balance and spiritual growth. By embracing yoga, seniors can unlock many benefits that contribute to a vibrant, healthy, and fulfilling later life.

Getting Started: Preparing for Your Yoga Journey

Embarking on a yoga journey, especially in later life, is a transformative step towards embracing a healthier, more balanced lifestyle. Whether new to yoga or returning after a break, beginning your practice under the right conditions is crucial for ensuring safety, enjoyment, and long-term commitment. Here are key steps and considerations to help you prepare for your yoga journey, making it both rewarding and sustainable.

Consult with Your Healthcare Provider
Before starting any new exercise regimen, it's essential to consult with your healthcare provider, particularly if you have existing health conditions, are recovering from surgery, or have mobility concerns. This step ensures that yoga is safe for you and helps identify any modifications you need to make to your practice.

Choose the Right Type of Yoga
Yoga comes in various styles, from gentle and restorative to more physically demanding types. For seniors or beginners, starting with gentler forms, such as Hatha or Chair Yoga, which focus on slow movements, foundational poses, and alignment, is advisable. Research or consult with yoga instructors to find a style that matches your physical capabilities and wellness goals.

Find a Qualified Yoga Instructor
A knowledgeable and experienced instructor is invaluable, especially when you're starting. Look for teachers with experience working with seniors or beginners, emphasizing safety and individual attention. Don't hesitate to ask about their training, knowledge, and approach to teaching yoga to individuals with varying abilities.

Create a Comfortable Space

Designate a quiet, comfortable space for your yoga practice. It doesn't need to be large, but it should be free from distractions and have enough room for you to move and stretch. Good ventilation and natural light can enhance the ambiance and your overall experience.

Start Slow and Set Realistic Goals

Begin your yoga journey with short, manageable sessions, gradually increasing duration and intensity as your comfort and confidence grow. Setting realistic goals, such as practicing a specific number of times per week, can help maintain motivation without causing strain or discouragement.

Listen to Your Body

One of the most critical aspects of yoga is developing an awareness of your body and its signals. Practice mindfulness and respect your body's limitations. If something feels painful or uncomfortable, adjust your pose or use props to find a variation that works for you. Remember, yoga is not a competition; it's a personal practice.

Embrace the Holistic Nature of Yoga

Yoga is more than just physical exercise; it's a holistic practice encompassing physical postures, breathing techniques, meditation, and lifestyle principles. Explore these different aspects to fully experience the benefits of yoga, including stress reduction, mental clarity, and a sense of inner peace.

Stay Consistent and Patient

Consistency is vital to experiencing yoga's full benefits. It may take time to notice significant changes, so be patient with yourself. Celebrate your progress, no matter how small, and remember that every step forward is a victory in your wellness journey.

By following these steps, you're well on your way to a fulfilling and enriching yoga practice. Yoga is a journey of discovery, not just about your physical abilities but also about your inner strength, resilience, and the joy of living a balanced life. Welcome to your yoga journey—may it bring you health, happiness, and profound well-being.

Assessing Your Current Health and Mobility

Before starting a yoga journey, assessing your health and mobility is crucial, especially for seniors. This evaluation will help you understand your starting point, allowing you to choose the most appropriate yoga practices and avoid injury. Here's a comprehensive guide on assessing your health and mobility, ensuring a safe and enjoyable yoga experience.

Consult with Healthcare Professionals

Medical Check-Up: Schedule an appointment with your healthcare provider for a general check-up. Discuss your intention to start yoga and any concerns you might have regarding your health conditions.

Specialist Advice: If you have specific health issues, such as heart problems, arthritis, or osteoporosis, consult specialists. They can provide tailored advice and precautions.

Self-Evaluation of Physical Health

Flexibility: Assess your flexibility by noting how easy or difficult it is to perform simple movements like bending forward, reaching overhead, or twisting your torso.

Balance: Test your balance by standing on one foot, then the other, with your eyes open and, if safe, closed. Assess how long you can hold the position without support.

Strength: Evaluate your strength by attempting basic exercises like sitting and rising from a chair without using your hands or holding a plank position for a few seconds.

Mobility Assessment

Range of Motion: Check the range of motion in your joints — shoulders, wrists, hips, knees, and ankles. Notice any stiffness or discomfort as you move them.

Daily Activities: Reflect on any difficulties you face with daily activities, such as walking, climbing stairs, or carrying groceries. These can indicate areas that need attention and improvement.

Pain and Discomfort Awareness

Identify any areas of chronic pain or discomfort. Be mindful of lower back pain, joint pain, or neck stiffness. Acknowledging these areas will help you approach yoga cautiously and adapt practices accordingly.

Cardiovascular Health

Assess your cardiovascular health by noting how you feel during and after moderate physical activity, such as brisk walking. Pay attention to your breathing, heart rate, and any signs of excessive fatigue.

Mental and Emotional Health

Reflect on your mental and emotional state. Yoga not only benefits the body but also the mind. Recognizing stress, anxiety, or depression is crucial, as yoga offers practices to help manage these conditions.

Setting Realistic Goals

Based on your assessment, set realistic health and mobility goals. Your goals will guide your yoga practice, whether improving flexibility, building strength, enhancing balance, or reducing stress.

Choosing the Right Yoga Style

With an understanding of your current health and mobility, select a yoga style that aligns with your needs. For example, Hatha or Iyengar yoga can be great for beginners due to their slower pace and emphasis on alignment. Chair yoga might be suitable for those with limited mobility.

Documenting Your Baseline

Keep a record of your initial health and mobility assessment. This documentation can be incredibly motivating as you track your progress over time, noticing the improvements yoga brings to your life.

Listening to Your Body

As you begin your yoga practice, continually listen to your body. Use your initial assessment as a guide, but remember that your abilities might vary daily. Adjust your practice accordingly, always prioritizing safety and comfort.

Assessing your current health and mobility is a vital first step in your yoga journey, paving the way for a practice that accommodates your needs and enhances your overall well-being. This mindful beginning ensures a rewarding experience with yoga tailored just for you.

Essential Yoga Gear for Seniors

Having the right gear can significantly improve comfort, safety, and overall enjoyment for seniors embarking on a yoga journey. Yoga doesn't require a lot of equipment, but a few essential items can help accommodate the needs of older practitioners, ensuring a fulfilling and injury-free experience. Here's a guide to the crucial yoga gear for seniors.

Yoga Mat

Thickness: A thicker mat (around 1/4 to 1/2 inch) provides extra cushioning for joints, which is beneficial for seniors who may have arthritis or sensitivity in the knees, wrists, or hips.

Texture and Material: Look for a mat with an excellent grip to prevent slipping. It is made of durable, eco-friendly material for long-lasting use.

Size: Ensure the mat is long and wide enough to fit your body and comfortably allow for various poses.

Yoga Blocks

Functionality: Blocks can modify poses, bringing the floor closer to you. They are excellent for maintaining balance and alignment, making poses more accessible.

Material: Foam blocks are lightweight and ideal for gentle use, while cork or wooden blocks offer more stability and support for heavier weight or more intensive practices.

Yoga Straps

Purpose: Straps help extend your reach, making it easier to grasp your feet, hands, or other limbs in stretches without straining. They're perfect for improving flexibility and safely deepening stretches.

Features: Look for a durable strap with an adjustable buckle to help secure it in loops or hold it at varying lengths.

Yoga Bolster

Use: A bolster can support the body in restorative poses, provide extra cushioning, and facilitate more profound relaxation. It's beneficial for seated or lying poses where additional support is desired.

Varieties: They come in different shapes and sizes (e.g., cylindrical, rectangular), so choose one that suits your body type and the practices you intend to do.

Comfortable Clothing

Requirements: Wear breathable, stretchy clothing that moves with you but isn't too loose-fitting, as overly baggy clothes can hinder movement or get caught during poses.

Layers: Consider layers that can be easily added or removed, accommodating changes in body temperature during and after practice.

Chair for Chair Yoga

Specifications: A sturdy, armless chair can be an excellent tool for those practicing chair yoga or needing extra support. Ensure the chair is stable and at a height that allows your feet to touch the ground comfortably.

Non-slip socks or Yoga Shoes

Option for Stability: For those who prefer not to practice barefoot, non-slip yoga socks or specially designed yoga shoes can provide additional grip, helping prevent slips and falls.

Water Bottle

Hydration: Keeping hydrated is crucial, especially for seniors. Have a water bottle handy to ensure you drink plenty of fluids before, during, and after your yoga session.

Yoga Towel

Absorbency: A yoga towel can be laid over your mat to absorb sweat and improve grip. This is particularly useful in more dynamic practices or if you tend to have sweaty palms.

Meditation Cushion or Bench

Support for Meditation: For those incorporating meditation into their yoga practice, a cushion or bench can provide comfortable seating, helping maintain proper posture and focus during meditation.

Investing in these essential items can significantly enhance the yoga experience for seniors, promoting safety, comfort, and the ability to engage with the practice entirely. Remember, yoga is about personal growth and well-being, so choose gear that best supports your needs and journey.

Creating a Safe and Comfortable Yoga Space

Creating a safe and comfortable yoga space is essential, particularly for seniors, as it sets the stage for a nurturing, effective, and enjoyable practice. Whether you're carving out a corner in your home or dedicating an entire room to yoga, the environment where you practice plays a crucial role in your yoga journey. Here's how to create a yoga space supporting your physical needs, inner peace, and well-being.

Choose the Right Location

Quiet and Private: Select a space where you're unlikely to be disturbed. This could be a spare room, a quiet corner of your bedroom, or a section of your living room.

Adequate Space: Ensure enough room for your yoga mat and any movements or poses you'll be doing. You should be able to stretch your arms and legs freely in all directions.

Ensure Proper Flooring

Stable Surface: Practice on a flat, stable surface to ensure balance and prevent injuries. Hardwood floors covered with a thick yoga mat or a low-pile carpet can provide stability and cushioning for joints.

Lighting and Ventilation

Natural Light: Choose a space with plenty of natural light if possible. It can enhance your mood and energy levels. However, make sure you can control the light intensity to avoid glare during your practice.

Good Ventilation: Fresh air is vital for keeping the space comfortable. Open windows for natural ventilation or use an air purifier to maintain air quality, especially if you're practicing in a smaller room.

Temperature Control

Comfortable Temperature: Keep the room cozy, neither too hot nor too cold. Depending on the season, this might mean adjusting your home's thermostat or using a portable heater or fan.

Minimize Distractions

Quiet Environment: Reduce noise distractions by turning off or muting electronic devices. You may also want to inform household members not to disturb you during practice.

Organized and Clutter-Free: Keep the space tidy and free from clutter. A clean, organized area promotes a calmer mind and more focused practice.

Personalize Your Space

Inspiring Elements: Add personal touches that inspire you or evoke peace and serenity. This could be anything from a small altar with meaningful items, plants for a touch of nature, or artwork that brings you joy.

Comfort Items: Consider including a few comfort items, such as cushions, blankets, or even a soft chair for meditation or relaxation before or after your practice.

Safety Features

Accessibility: Ensure your yoga space is easily accessible, especially if mobility concerns you. Avoid areas where you must navigate stairs or obstacles to your practice space.

Supportive Props: Have your yoga mat, blocks, straps, and other supportive props within easy reach to help balance and modify poses.

Creating Ambiance

Soothing Sounds: If you need to relax and focus, play soft, soothing music or natural sounds through a speaker or phone.

Aromatherapy: To enhance your sensory experience, incorporate calming scents using essential oil diffusers or candles (be mindful of fire safety).

Creating a yoga space that feels safe, comfortable, and uniquely yours can significantly enhance the benefits of your practice. This personalized sanctuary supports your physical training and nurtures your mental and emotional well-being, making yoga a gratifying part of your daily routine.

Chapter II

The Power of Pranayama: Breathing Exercises for Vitality

Pranayama, the practice of breath control in yoga, is a powerful tool for enhancing physical health, mental clarity, and emotional balance. This ancient practice involves various techniques to increase vitality, reduce stress, and improve the overall quality of life. Here are several pranayama exercises that are especially beneficial for cultivating vitality and well-being. These exercises suit all levels, including beginners and seniors, and can be easily integrated into your daily routine.

Deep Abdominal Breathing (Diaphragmatic Breathing)
Benefits: Reduces stress, lowers blood pressure, improves core muscle stability, and increases lung capacity.
How to Do: Sit or lie down in a comfortable position. Place one hand on your chest and the other on your belly. Breathe slowly through your nose, allowing your belly to rise more than your chest. Exhale slowly through your mouth or nose, engaging your abdominal muscles to empty your lungs. Repeat for 5-10 minutes.

Three-Part Breath (Dirga Pranayama)
Benefits: Enhances lung capacity, reduces anxiety, and improves focus.
How to Do: Sit comfortably with your back straight. Begin by inhaling deeply, filling your abdomen, then your ribcage, and finally, your chest. Exhale in reverse order: chest, ribcage, and stomach. Use smooth, flowing breaths without pausing between the inhalation and exhalation. Practice for 5-10 cycles.

Alternate Nostril Breathing (Nadi Shodhana Pranayama)
Benefits: Balances the left and right hemispheres of the brain, calms the mind, reduces stress, and improves cardiovascular function.
How to Do: Sit in a comfortable position with your spine straight. Rest your left hand on your knee. Use your right hand to close your right nostril with your thumb. Inhale through your left nostril, then close it with your fingers. Open your right nostril and exhale. Inhale through the right nostril, close it, and exhale through the left. This completes one cycle. Continue for 5-10 cycles.

Bee Breath (Bhramari Pranayama)
Benefits: Instantly calms the mind, relieves tension and anger, and reduces blood pressure.
How to Do: Sit comfortably with your eyes closed. Cover your ears with your thumbs and place your fingers over your eyes. Take a deep breath through your nose, and as you exhale, make a loud humming sound like a bee. Repeat 5-10 times.

<u>*Lion's Breath (Simhasana Pranayama)*</u>
<u>Benefits:</u> Relieves stress and tension in the face and chest, improves circulation, and stimulates the throat and respiratory system.

How to Do: Sit comfortably with your palms on your knees, fingers spread wide. Inhale through the nose, and as you exhale, open your mouth wide, stick out your tongue towards your chin, and make a "ha" sound from deep within your abdomen. Repeat 3-5 times.

Practice Tips for Pranayama

Consistency: Regular practice yields the best results. Aim to incorporate pranayama into your daily routine, even for a few minutes.

Comfortable Setting: Practice in a quiet, comfortable place where you won't be disturbed.

Posture: Maintain a comfortable seated position with an erect spine for optimal breathing.

Mindfulness: Focus on your breath and the sensations it brings. This mindfulness aspect enhances the benefits of pranayama.

Progress Gradually: Start with more straightforward techniques, and as you become more comfortable, explore more advanced breathing exercises.

Pranayama is a critical component of yoga that extends beyond physical health, offering a pathway to deeper self-awareness and inner peace. By practicing these breathing exercises, you can unlock the door to enhanced vitality and a more balanced state of being.

Meditation Techniques for Stress Relief and Clarity

Meditation is a powerful tool for alleviating stress, fostering mental clarity, and promoting emotional well-being. Various techniques can suit different preferences and goals, making meditation accessible to everyone. Here are several effective meditation methods focused on reducing stress and enhancing clarity.

Mindfulness Meditation
Practice: Sit comfortably with your eyes closed or gaze lowered and focus on your breath. Observe your thoughts, feelings, and sensations as they arise without judgment or attachment. When your mind wanders, gently bring your attention back to your breath.

<u>Benefits:</u> Increases awareness of the present moment, reduces stress, and enhances emotional balance.

Body Scan Meditation
Practice: Lie down or sit comfortably. Focus on each body part, starting at your feet and moving to your head. Notice any sensations, tension, or discomfort without trying to change anything. Use your breath to release tension as you move through your body.

<u>Benefits:</u> Relaxes the body, reduces physical tension and stress, and improves body awareness.

Loving-Kindness Meditation (Metta Bhavana)

Practice: Begin by focusing on yourself and generating feelings of kindness and compassion. Mentally repeat phrases like "May I be happy, may I be healthy, may I be safe, may I live with ease." Gradually extend these wishes to loved ones, acquaintances, and even those you struggle with.

Benefits: Promotes feelings of compassion and empathy, decreases stress and anxiety, and improves interpersonal relationships.

Guided Visualization

Practice: Listen to a guided meditation recording where you're led through a series of relaxing images or scenarios. Focus on the details of these visualizations, immersing yourself in the experience.

Benefits: Eases stress, enhances mood, and fosters creativity and problem-solving abilities.

Breath Awareness Meditation

Practice: Sit or lie comfortably and focus on your natural breathing pattern. Please pay attention to the sensation of the breath as it enters and leaves your nostrils or the rise and fall of your chest or abdomen.

Benefits: Calms the mind, reduces stress, and improves concentration and mindfulness.

Mantra Meditation

Practice: Choose a word, phrase, or sound to focus on. Repeat your mantra silently or aloud, allowing it to help you focus and quiet the mind. When distractions arise, gently return your attention to your mantra.

Benefits: Reduces stress and anxiety, centers the mind, and promotes peace and focus.

Walking Meditation

Practice: Find a quiet path or area to walk slowly and deliberately. Focus on the sensation of walking, noticing the movement of your feet and the sensations in your body with each step. Use your breath to help you maintain focus and rhythm.

Benefits: Engages the body and mind, reduces stress, and increases mindfulness in everyday activities.

Tips for Effective Meditation Practice

Consistency: Regular practice, even for just a few minutes a day, can significantly enhance the benefits of meditation.

Comfort: During meditation, ensure you're comfortable and free from distractions. Use cushions, chairs, or any supportive props you need.

Patience: Be patient with yourself. Meditation is a skill that develops over time, and it's normal for the mind to wander.

Experiment: Try different techniques to find what works best for you. Meditation is a personal journey, and there's no one-size-fits-all approach.

Incorporating meditation into your daily routine can be a transformative practice for managing stress, gaining clarity, and cultivating a more profound sense of inner peace.

Incorporating Mindfulness into Your Yoga Practice

Incorporating mindfulness into your yoga practice can transform it from a series of physical exercises into a profoundly enriching, holistic experience that nurtures the mind, body, and spirit. Mindfulness in yoga involves paying deliberate, nonjudgmental attention to your movements, breath, and sensations in the present moment. Here's how you can weave mindfulness into your yoga routine to deepen your practice and enhance its benefits.

Set an Intention (Sankalpa)
Start with Intention: Begin each yoga session by setting an intention. This could be a word or phrase that resonates with you, such as peace, gratitude, or strength. Let this intention guide your practice, bringing your focus back to it whenever your mind wanders.

Start with Pranayama
Please use any pranayama technique that is most requested or favored today.
Breath as an Anchor: Use your breath as a focal point throughout your practice. Observe the rhythm of your breath, its depth, and how it feels as you move through poses. Breathing mindfully helps anchor you in the present moment and enhances the connection between mind and body.

Practice Active Observation
Observe Without Judgment: Pay attention to your body's sensations during each pose. Notice areas of tension or ease without judgment. If you encounter discomfort, observe it with curiosity rather than resistance. This observation practice lets you connect more deeply with your body's needs and limitations.

Move with Awareness
Conscious Movement: Execute each movement with full awareness, as if you're experiencing it for the first time. Be mindful of how you transition from one pose to another, focusing on your breath and the sensations in your body.

Embrace Stillness
Find Stillness in Poses: Allow yourself to be still in each pose, even if it's uncomfortable or challenging. Stillness in practice fosters mental clarity and calmness. Use this time to observe your breath and any sensations or emotions that arise.

Cultivate Self-Compassion
Be Kind to Yourself: Approach your practice with kindness and compassion. Recognize and honor your body's strengths and limitations on any given day. Remember, yoga is not about achieving the perfect pose but the journey toward self-awareness and acceptance.

Integrate Mindfulness Off the Mat
Carry Mindfulness Into Daily Life: Extend the mindfulness cultivated during your yoga practice into your daily activities, whether eating, walking, or listening to someone and practice being fully present. This continuity of mindfulness can profoundly impact your overall well-being.

End with Reflection
Reflect on Your Practice: Conclude your session with a few minutes of quiet reflection or meditation. Consider what you observed about your body, mind, and emotions during practice. Acknowledge and appreciate your efforts, and revisit the intention you set at the beginning.

Incorporating mindfulness into your yoga practice can significantly enhance its benefits, leading to more excellent emotional balance, mental clarity, and physical well-being. By practicing with intention, awareness, and compassion, you deepen your connection to the present moment, cultivating peace and contentment beyond the mat.

Postures of Peace: The Essence of Asana in Yoga

Asana refers to the physical postures or poses in yoga designed to purify the body and provide the physical strength and stamina required for long periods of meditation. The term "asana" comes from the Sanskrit word meaning "seat" or "manner of sitting." However, in the context of yoga, it extends beyond sitting postures to encompass a variety of physical positions.
Asanas are vital to yoga. They serve physical health benefits and prepare the mind and body for pranayama (breathing exercises) and meditation. Each asana targets specific muscles, organs, or systems within the body, promoting strength, flexibility, and physical and mental balance. Regular practice of asanas can improve digestion, circulation, and posture, reduce stress, and enhance concentration and emotional well-being.
Hundreds of asanas range from simple poses like Tadasana (Mountain Pose) to more complex ones like Sirsasana (Headstand). The practice of asanas is not about achieving perfect form but rather about exploring the limits of one's body and mind and learning to move with breath and awareness.

Harmonizing Energy: The Vibrant Journey Through the Chakras with Yoga

Yoga and the chakras are intertwined in a beautiful dance of energy and physicality, bridging our bodies' tangible world and the intangible essence of our spiritual selves. This connection is fundamental to how yoga can lead to deeper self-awareness, balance, and healing.
The chakras, seven energy centers along the spine, each correspond to different aspects of our physical, emotional, and spiritual well-being. From the root chakra, which grounds us to

the Earth, to the crown chakra, which connects us to the divine, each chakra plays a crucial role in our health and vitality.

Yoga offers a direct pathway to engage with and balance these energy centers with its wide variety of poses (asanas), breathwork (pranayama), and meditation techniques. Through asanas, we can stimulate and open up blocked or stagnant areas within our body, allowing energy (prana) to flow freely. Pranayama practices help to channel this energy further, clearing the pathways (nadis) and awakening the chakras. Meditation brings awareness and harmony to the mind and spirit, aligning the chakras in a symphony of balance and enlightenment.

By understanding the connection between specific yoga practices and the chakras they influence, practitioners can intentionally address issues such as insecurity, creativity blockages, lack of confidence, heartache, communication difficulties, vision clarity, and spiritual disconnect. For instance, grounding asanas may help to stabilize an unbalanced root chakra, while heart-opening poses can nurture an underactive heart chakra, fostering love and compassion.

Incorporating chakra awareness into yoga enhances physical flexibility and strength and fosters inner peace, emotional resilience, and a more profound sense of connection to the universe. This holistic approach empowers individuals to navigate life's challenges gracefully and embrace their journey with an open heart and a clear mind.

Thus, the symbiotic relationship between yoga and the chakras is a testament to the profound layers of healing and growth accessible to those who embark on this transformative path. Through this integration, we can tap into our most profound potential, unlocking a wellspring of vitality, creativity, and spiritual enlightenment that enriches our lives in every way.

Embarking on a journey through the chakras is like opening the door to the deeper dimensions of well-being, especially for seniors who seek balance, vitality, and a renewed sense of being in their later years. This upcoming section of our book, "Yoga for Seniors," invites you to explore the fascinating world of chakras, the seven energy centers along the spine that influence physical, emotional, and spiritual health.

Each day, we will dedicate our practice to one of the seven chakras, starting from the root and ascending to the crown. This approach allows us to focus on specific areas of our lives and bodies that each chakra represents, promoting a holistic balance that enhances well-being at all levels.

For each chakra, we incorporate a holistic approach to our practice that encompasses four key elements tailored to be accessible and beneficial for seniors:

Pranayama Breathing involves using specific breathing techniques designed to enhance energy flow in and around the chakras, facilitating balance and healing.

Affirmation: We introduce a positive affirmation for each chakra. These affirmations are powerful statements that reinforce the qualities and energies we aim to cultivate, strengthening our mental and emotional health.

Asanas: We select specific yoga poses that are particularly effective in stimulating and balancing each chakra. These poses are chosen for their accessibility to seniors, ensuring everyone can participate safely and gain the full benefits.

Mindfulness Practice: Simple mindfulness techniques are integrated to bring awareness to the present moment. This practice fosters a deep connection between body, mind, and spirit, enhancing overall well-being and tranquility.

By weaving these elements into our daily routines, we enhance our physical flexibility and strength and embark on a profound journey of inner transformation. This journey through the chakras helps to unlock energy blockages, promote healing, and awaken a deeper understanding of our true selves. Through this integrated practice, we aim to achieve a harmonious balance that resonates throughout our lives.

As we progress from the Root Chakra's grounding energy to the Crown Chakra's divine illumination, we invite you to open your heart and mind to the transformative power of this ancient wisdom. Let's embrace this journey with patience, curiosity, and compassion, discovering the infinite possibilities within us.

Understanding the Chakras

The word "chakra" translates to "wheel" in Sanskrit, symbolizing the dynamic interplay of energy within us. These spinning wheels of energy correspond to nerve centers in the body and are thought to influence our physical, emotional, mental, and spiritual health.

There are seven main chakras, each located along the spine, from the base to the crown of the head. Each chakra governs specific bodily functions and embodies distinct aspects of our being and life experiences. Here is a brief overview:

Root Chakra (Muladhara):
The foundation of the chakra system, located at the base of the spine, represents our sense of security, survival, and belonging.

Sacral Chakra (Svadhishthana):
 Positioned just below the navel, this chakra governs our emotions, creativity, and sexual energy.

Solar Plexus Chakra (Manipura):
Located in the abdomen, it influences our power, self-esteem, and ability to assert ourselves.

Heart Chakra (Anahata):
Situated in the chest, it's the center of love, compassion, and connection with others and the self.

Throat Chakra (Vishuddha):
Positioned at the throat, it encompasses communication, self-expression, and the ability to speak our truth.

Third Eye Chakra (Ajna):
Located between the eyebrows, it relates to intuition, insight, and the ability to see beyond the superficial.

Crown Chakra (Sahasrara):
It connects us to the divine at the top of the head, representing spiritual awakening and enlightenment.

Working with the chakras aims to achieve a balance, allowing energy to flow freely throughout the body. An imbalance in a chakra can lead to physical, emotional, or spiritual disturbances. Through various practices such as yoga, meditation, pranayama (breath work), and lifestyle adjustments, one can work towards harmonizing each chakra, thereby promoting overall well-being.

As we delve deeper into the chakra system, we embark on self-discovery, healing, and transformation. This journey is not linear but a continuous exploration of our inner landscape, revealing the interconnectedness of our physical, emotional, mental, and spiritual layers. Through awareness and practice, we can navigate the challenges and joys of life with greater ease, harmony, and fulfillment.

Chapter III
Journey to Inner Harmony: A Transformative Yoga Practice

Embarking on a morning yoga practice can set a positive tone for your day, promoting clarity, calmness, and intention. As an experienced yoga practitioner, I've designed a comprehensive morning yoga routine encompassing affirmations, a calming atmosphere, setting intentions (Sankalpa), and integrating the Om (AUM) mantra to create a holistic practice. Here's a detailed guide to starting your day with purpose and serenity through yoga.

Setting the Stage for Practice

Create a Calming Space: Choose a quiet, comfortable spot for your practice where you won't be disturbed. You might want to include elements like a yoga mat, cushions, or a blanket and possibly light a candle or incense to create a serene atmosphere.

Begin with Centering:

Start in a comfortable seated position, either in Lotus (Padmasana) or Simple Cross-Legged Pose (Sukhasana). In a prayer pose, bring your palms together in front of your heart, closing your eyes gently. Feel the warmth between your palms, and center your awareness on your breath. Allow yourself to arrive fully in the present moment, setting aside thoughts of the day ahead.

Mantra:

Choose a mantra to chant, such as "Om" or "So Hum," to deepen your focus and connection to your practice. During mantra chanting, listen closely to feel the vibration within you.

Incorporating Affirmations:

Choose Your Affirmation: Begin by selecting an affirmation for your practice. This could be a positive statement that resonates with your current intentions, such as "I am grounded and serene" or "Today, I choose joy."

Integrate with Breath:

Please use any pranayama technique that is most requested or favored today.

With each inhalation, silently repeat your affirmation to yourself, allowing its energy to fill you. With each exhalation, release any doubts or negativity.

Setting a Sankalpa (Intention):

Formulate Your Sankalpa: Reflect on a deeper intention for your practice, something that speaks to your higher goals or desires, such as cultivating patience, kindness, or a sense of gratitude, something that resonates with your deepest desires and values.

Internalize Your Sankalpa:

Hold your Sankalpa in your heart as you breathe deeply, envisioning it taking root within you, guiding your practice and your actions throughout the day.

Asana Practice:

Warming up before yoga is crucial to enhancing your body's flexibility and performance while significantly reducing the risk of injury. A warm-up gradually increases the heart rate, blood flow to the muscles, and body temperature, making the muscles more elastic and receptive to stretching and movement. It also helps to mentally prepare for the practice, allowing for a transition from the hustle and bustle of daily life to a more reflective and mindful state.

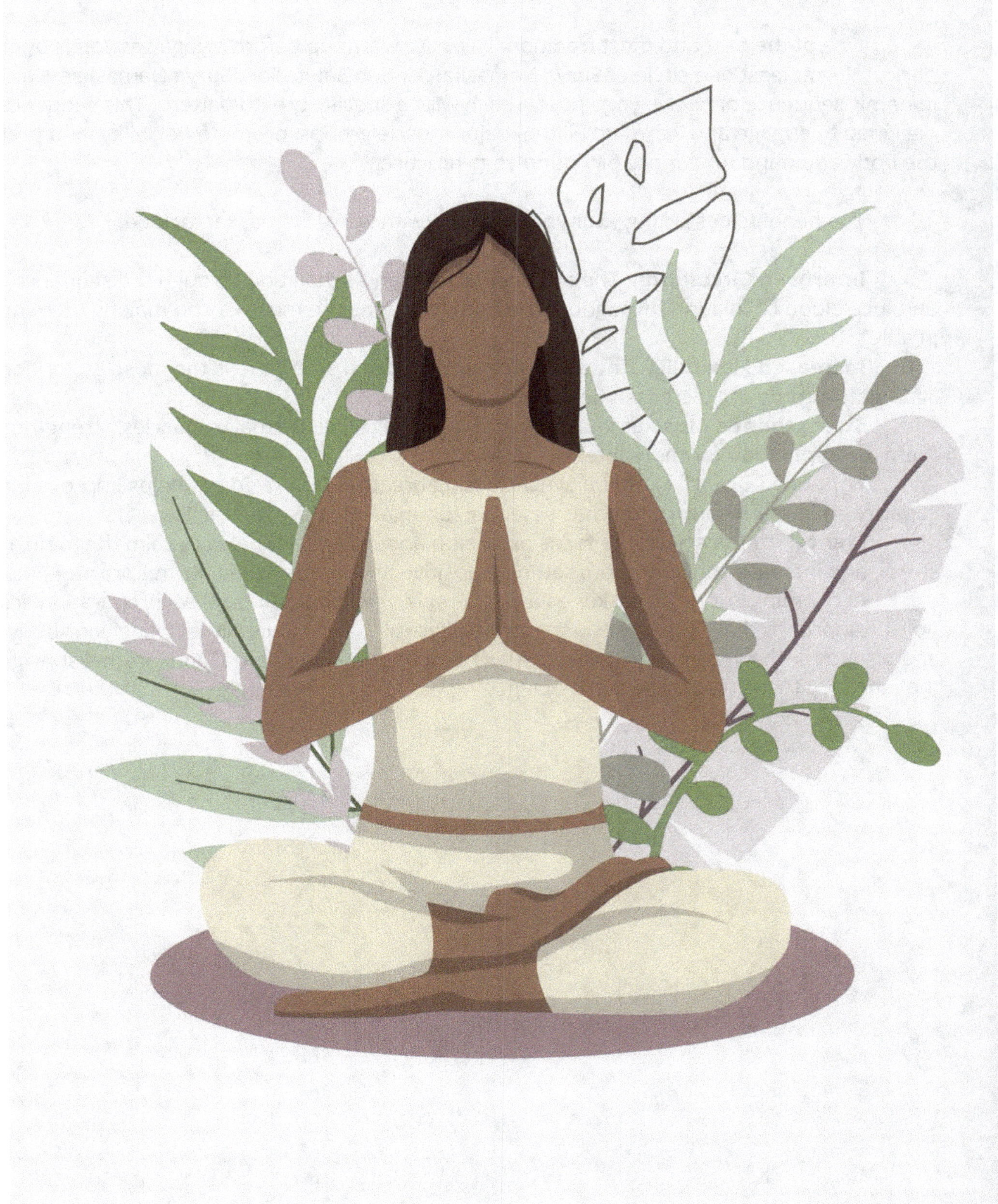

Exploring Surya Namaskar: A Comprehensive Guide to Sun Salutation

One of the best and most traditional ways to warm up before a yoga session is by performing at least one circle of Surya Namaskar, or Sun Salutation. Surya Namaskar is a dynamic sequence of twelve yoga poses, each with a specific breath pattern. This sequence is designed to engage and warm up all the major muscle groups, promote flexibility, and prepare the body and mind for a more profound yoga practice.

The benefits of starting your yoga practice with Surya Namaskar include:

Improved Circulation: The active inhalation and exhalation through the sequence enhance blood circulation throughout the body, warming the muscles and making them more pliable.

Increased Flexibility: The sequence stretches and strengthens the muscles, tendons, and ligaments, promoting increased flexibility.

Strengthened Muscles: Surya Namaskar engages all the major muscles, strengthening them as preparation for more intense poses.

Enhanced Breath Control: Synchronizing breath with movement helps improve lung capacity and breath control, which is essential for an effective yoga practice.

Mental Preparation: The focus on breath and movement helps to calm the mind, reduce stress, and increase concentration, setting a positive and mindful tone for the practice.

Performing Surya Namaskar as a warm-up is not just about physical preparation; it's a holistic approach that prepares you mentally, physically, and spiritually, aligning your body, mind, and breath for the yoga practice ahead. This ritual honors the external and internal sun, igniting the inner fire (Agni) that powers our being.

12 steps of Surya Namaskar

Below you will find an overview of the 12 steps of Surya Namaskar, complete with pictures and clear instructions for each pose's technique and process. Additionally, the benefits and mantras associated with each step can be chanted to reap the full rewards of each yoga pose in the Surya Namaskar sequence.

This structured approach helps beginners understand and practice Surya Namaskar effectively, ensuring a balanced and enriching yoga experience.

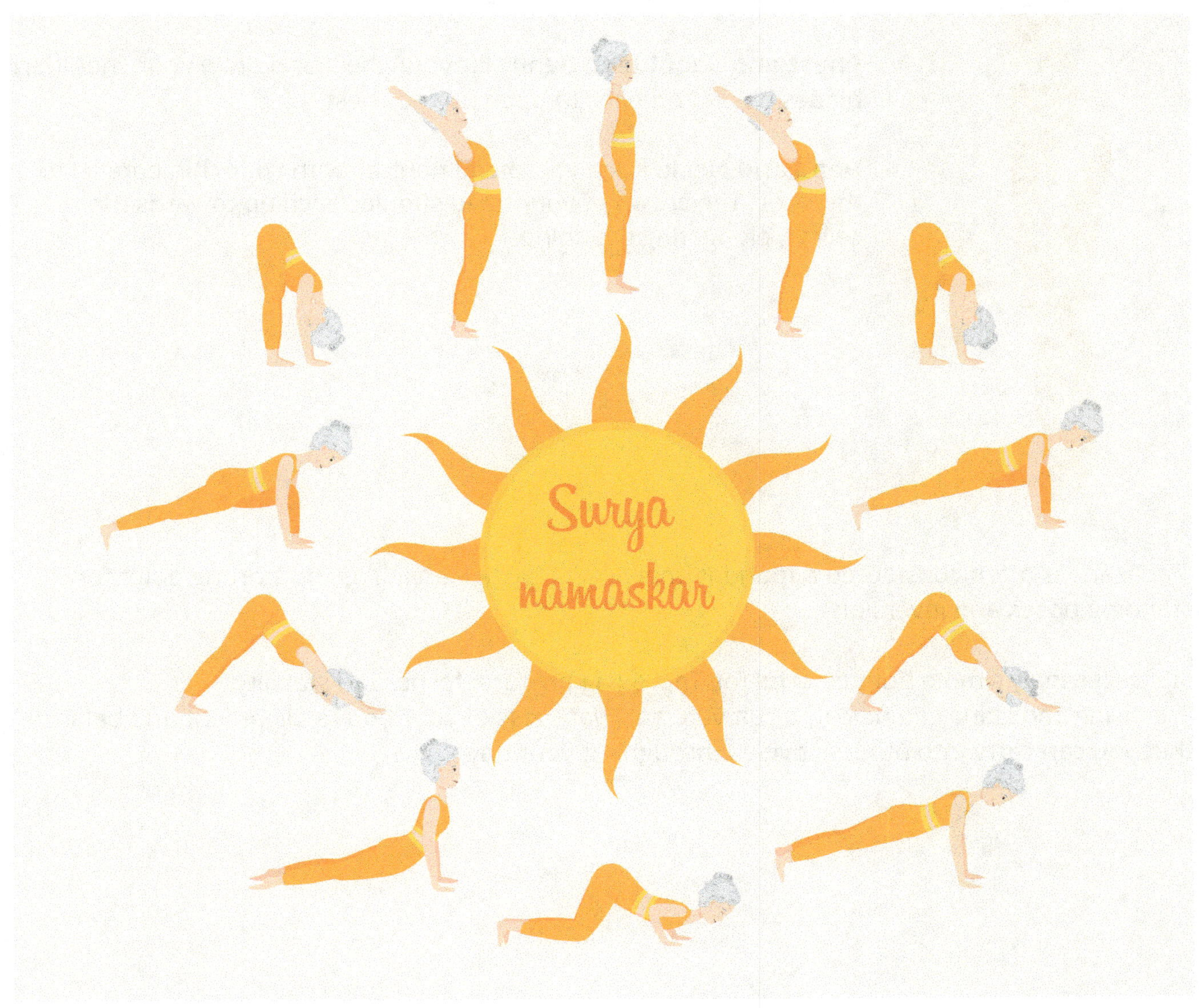

Tadasana (Mountain Pose)

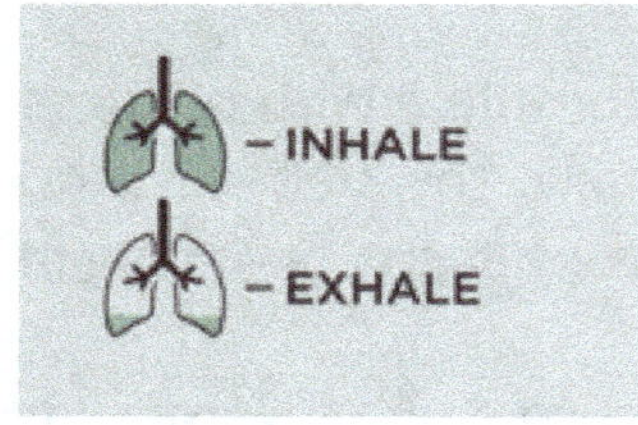

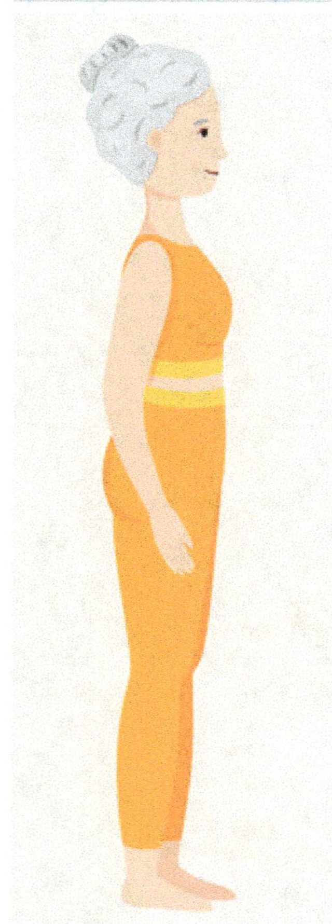

Standard Pose:

Position: Stand with your feet together, heels slightly apart, or hip-width apart for more stability. Distribute your weight evenly across the balls and heels of both feet.

Alignment: Align your body so that your ears, shoulders, hips, and ankles are in a straight line. Engage your thigh muscles slightly to lift your kneecaps, but don't lock your knees.

Arms: Let your arms rest at your sides with fingers together and palms facing your body. Feel as though you are stretching your arms downwards.

Chest and Shoulders: Gently lift your chest and draw your shoulder blades down and back to open up the chest.

Head and Neck: Keep your head neutral, with your chin parallel to the floor. The crown of your head should reach up towards the ceiling, elongating the spine.

Tadasana is often considered a foundational pose in yoga, serving as the starting point for standing poses and inversions.

It's deceivingly simple but powerful for improving posture, focus, and stability.
Practicing Tadasana can help you cultivate an awareness of your body's alignment and balance that you can carry into other activities throughout your day.

Hasta Uttanasana (Raised Arms Pose)

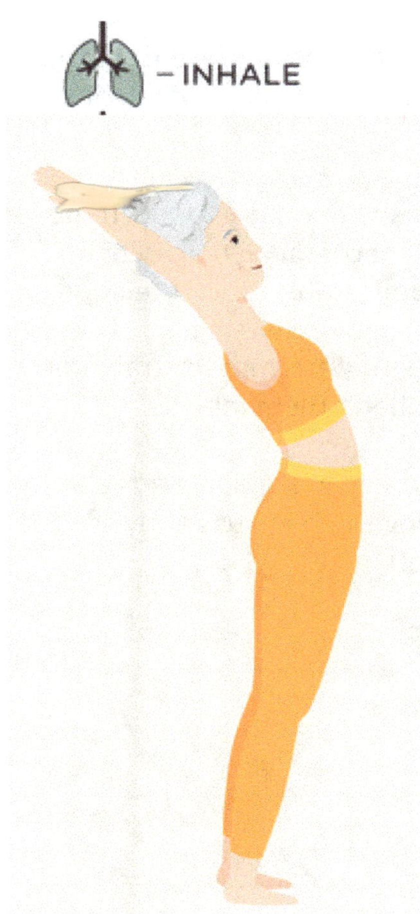

Arm Lift: Inhale and lift your arms up, keeping your biceps close to your ears.

Hip Alignment: Slightly push your hips forward to align correctly.

Body Stretch: Focus on stretching your entire body up from the heels to the tips of your fingers.

Upward Focus: Ensure your effort is on reaching up with your fingers rather than bending backward.

Stability: Stand firm and relaxed in this position.

Modification:
If raising arms ultimately is challenging, reach as high as comfortable. Alternatively, keep hands on hips if shoulder issues are present.

Benefits of Hasta Uttanasana:

Abdominal Stretch: Hasta Uttanasana stretches and tones the abdominal muscles, enhancing core strength.

Chest Expansion: It expands the chest, leading to increased oxygen intake.

Lung Capacity: Maximizes the use of lung capacity, promoting better breathing and improving respiratory function.

Incorporating Hasta Uttanasana into your Surya Namaskar practice offers a moment of energizing stretch and invigoration. It prepares the body for the sequence ahead by warming up the core, enhancing flexibility, and promoting a deep connection with the breath. This pose embodies the essence of greeting the sun - reaching upwards and outwards, embracing the energy and warmth of life.

Hasta Padasana (Standing Forward Bend)

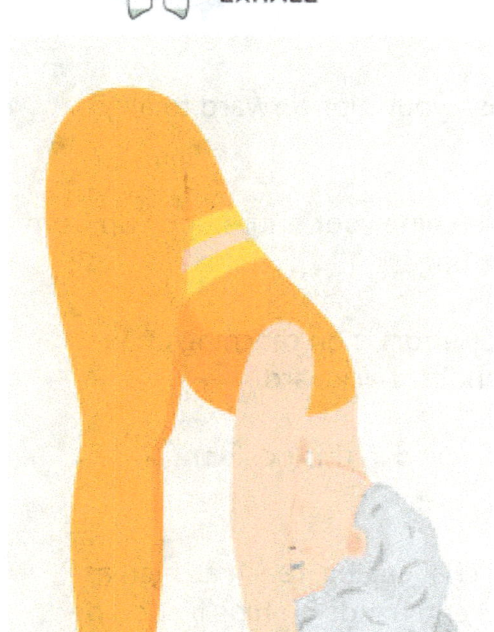

Forward Bend: Exhale and bend forward from the waist, ensuring that your spine remains straight as you fold.

Floor Touch: On a full exhalation, try to touch the floor next to your feet. If necessary, you can bend your knees slightly to comfortably touch the floor.

Knee Straightening: Gently attempt to straighten the knees if you have to bend them initially.

Stability and Relaxation: Find stability and relax into this position, allowing the body to gently stretch further with each exhalation.

Benefits of Hasta Padasana:

Flexibility: Hasta Padasana enhances flexibility in the waist and spine, promoting spinal health.

Hamstring Stretch: It stretches the hamstrings, aiding in the reduction of stiffness and improving leg flexibility.

Hip, Shoulder, and Arm Opening: The pose opens up the hips, shoulders, and arms, contributing to overall mobility and flexibility.

Incorporating Hasta Padasana into your Surya Namaskar routine offers an excellent opportunity to deepen your forward bends, promoting flexibility and opening the body. It serves as a grounding moment in the sequence, allowing for a deep inward turn and connection with the breath, preparing the practitioner for the subsequent poses with a sense of calm and centeredness.

Modifiication for Seniors

Use a Chair for Support:
Place a chair in front of you and bend forward from the hips, resting your hands on the chair seat. This modification reduces the distance you need to bend and provides stability, making it easier to maintain balance.
If necessary, adjust the chair's height or use a higher platform, like a table, to further reduce the bend.

Bend Knees Slightly:
Softening the knees during a forward bend can significantly reduce the strain on the lower back and hamstrings. This adjustment makes the pose more comfortable, especially if you have tight hamstrings or lower back issues.

Use Yoga Blocks:
Place yoga blocks on the ground before you to bring the floor closer. You can rest your hands on the blocks instead of reaching the floor. You can adjust the height of the blocks according to your comfort level.
This tool is beneficial for maintaining good alignment and reducing strain.

Wall Supported:
Stand facing a wall, step back about two feet, then hinge at the hips to press your hands into the wall. Keep your hands at hip height or lower to find a comfortable stretch. This version supports the upper body and can help maintain balance.

Hands-on Shins:
Instead of reaching for the floor, place your hands on your shins or just above your knees. Bend forward only as much as comfortable, keeping your back flat. This modification reduces the intensity of the stretch while still providing the benefits of the forward bend.

Hip-Width Stance:
Instead of keeping the feet together, seniors can stand with their feet hip-width apart or even more comprehensively for better balance and support. This stance provides a more stable base and can help distribute the stretch more comfortably across the lower back and legs.

These modifications help seniors practice Hasta Padasana safely, allowing them to gain the pose's benefits—such as stretching the spine and hamstrings, stimulating the abdominal organs, and calming the mind—without overstraining their bodies.

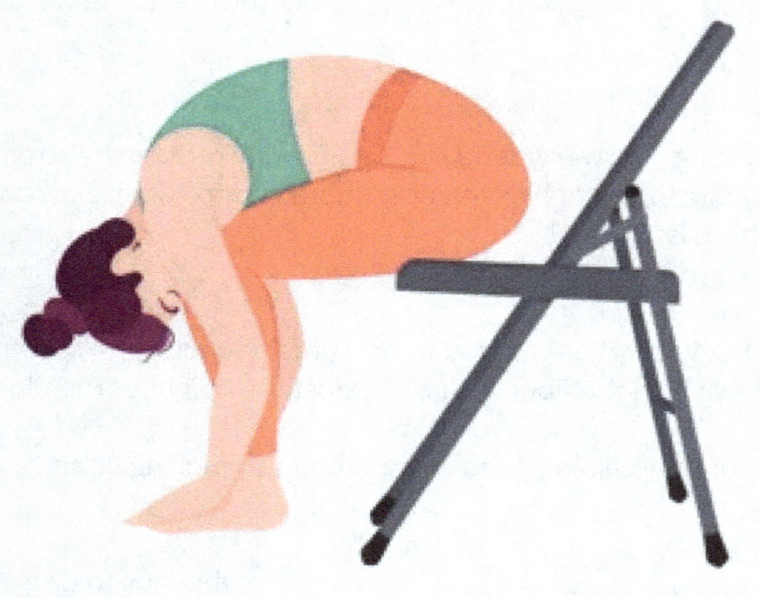

SEATED FORWARD BEND

Ashwa Sanchalanasana (Equestrian Pose)

Leg Position: Inhale and extend your right leg as far back as possible.

Knee Support: Rest your right knee on the ground.

Upper Body Stretch: While experiencing a stretch in your arms, hamstrings, and back, direct your gaze upwards towards the ceiling.

Front Leg Alignment: Ensure your left leg is perpendicular to the ground, positioned directly between your hands.

Palm Placement: Both palms should fully contact the floor, providing stability.

Steadiness and Relaxation: Maintain stability in this pose and relax into the position.

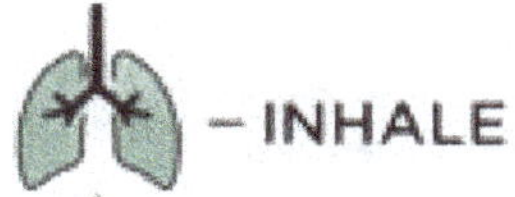

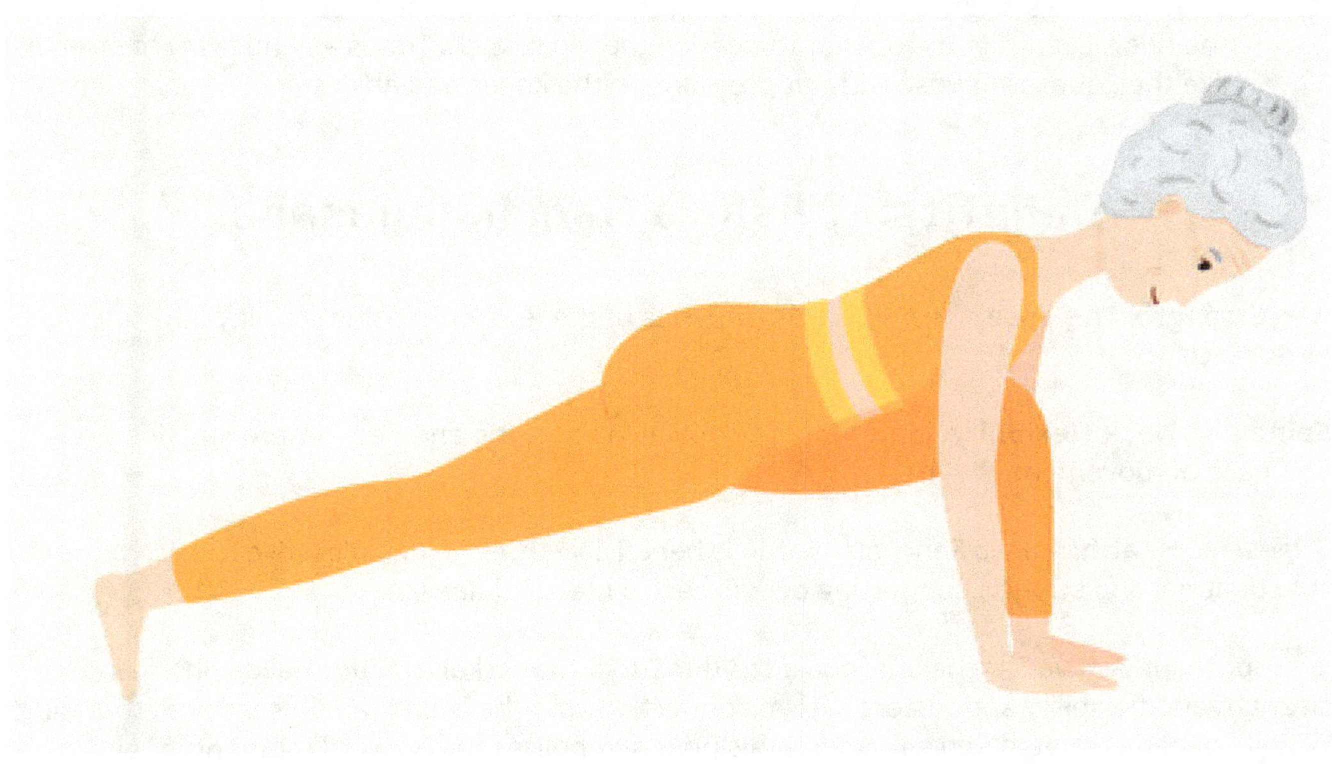

Modification for Seniors:

Use Props:

- **Yoga Blocks:** Place yoga blocks on either side of the front foot to rest your hands. This helps maintain balance and reduces strain on the hips and lower back.
- Chair Support: Perform the pose with the front foot forward and hands placed on the back of a sturdy chair. This provides support and stability while allowing for a comfortable hip stretch.

Cushion Under Back Knee:

- Place a folded blanket or a cushion under the back knee for extra padding, especially if kneeling on the floor is uncomfortable.

Standing Variation:

- Instead of performing the pose on the floor, do a standing version by stepping one foot forward and bending the front knee while keeping the back leg straight. Use a wall or a chair for support as needed. This variation helps stretch the hip flexors and strengthen the legs without kneeling.

Half Lunge with a Chair:

- Sit on a chair and slide to the edge. Extend one leg backward with the toe on the floor and the knee straight while the other leg remains bent at the knee with the foot flat on the floor. Lean slightly forward to deepen the hip stretch. This is a gentle way to stretch like the Equestrian Pose without pressure on the knees and ankles.

Benefits of Ashwa Sanchalanasana:

Leg Strength: This pose strengthens the muscles of the legs, enhancing stability and endurance.

Spine and Neck Flexibility: It promotes flexibility in the spine and neck, improving posture and ease of movement.

Digestive Health: Ashwa Sanchalanasana is beneficial for alleviating digestive issues, constipation, and sciatica, supporting overall gastrointestinal health.

Incorporating Ashwa Sanchalanasana into your Surya Namaskar practice builds physical strength and flexibility and fosters a deep connection with the breath and a sense of grounding. With its dynamic stretch and alignment, this pose symbolizes the forward momentum and vitality that embody the essence of the sun salutation sequence.

Adho Mukha Svanasana
(Downward-Facing Dog Pose)

Spread your fingers wide and press firmly through your palms.

Extend your spine and push your hips back.

Walk your feet hip-width apart, keeping them parallel. Your toes should point straight ahead. Initially, you can slightly bend your knees to ease into the pose.

Gradually try to straighten your legs, but don't lock your knees. It's okay if your heels don't touch the floor; flexibility will improve with practice.

Press into your palms and keep your arms straight. Rotate your arms externally to broaden your shoulders. Ensure your neck is long and your ears align with your inner arms.

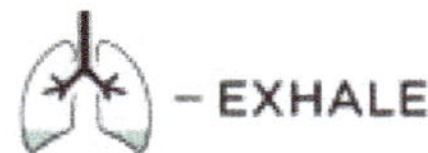 – EXHALE

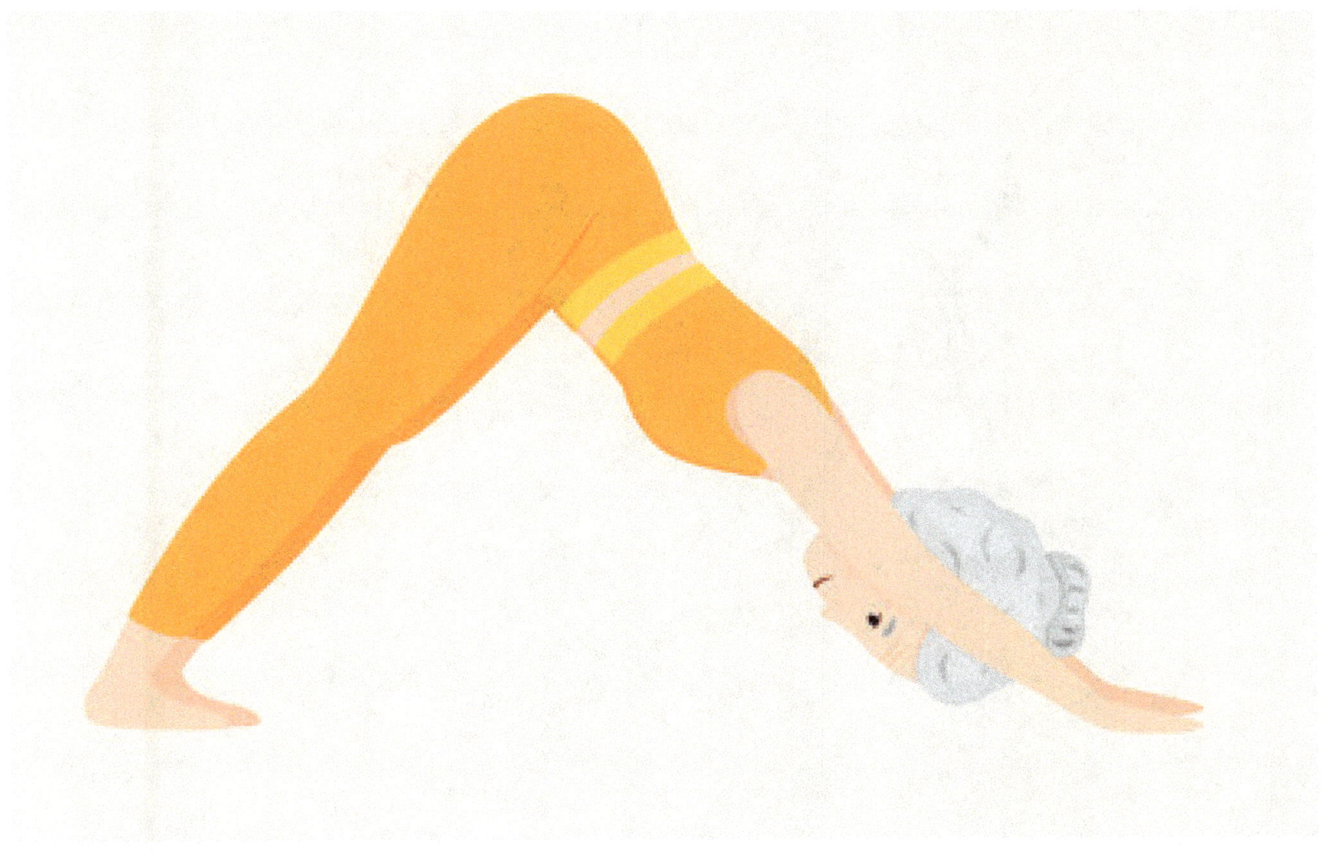

Modifications for Seniors:

Use a Chair: Place your hands on the seat of a chair instead of the floor. This reduces the angle of your body and the load on your arms and shoulders.

Elevate Your Hands: Use yoga blocks, a low stool, or the seat of a chair to elevate your hands. This helps lessen the intensity of the stretch and can be easier on your shoulders and wrists.

Keep Knees Bent: Maintain a slight knee bend to reduce the strain on the hamstrings and lower back.

Wall Support: Stand facing a wall, place your hands on the wall at waist height, and walk your feet back until your body forms a right angle. This "standing downward dog" variant reduces pressure on the wrists and shoulders while providing many of the same benefits.

Focus on Upper Body: If getting down to the floor is difficult, you can perform the pose with your hands placed on a kitchen counter, allowing the spine to elongate and the shoulders to open without the full inversion.

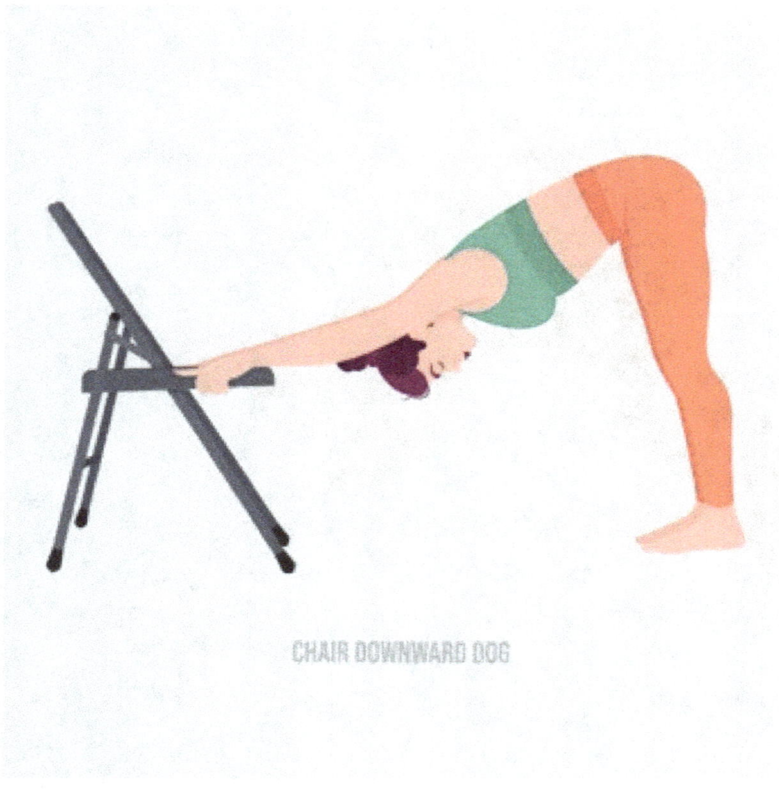

Benefits of practicing Downward-Facing Dog Pose

Physical Benefits:

Strengthens the Upper Body: The pose requires bearing weight on the arms and shoulders, which helps strengthen these areas along with the chest and upper back.

Stretches the Hamstrings and Calves: By extending the hips upwards and pressing the heels towards the floor, Downward-Facing Dog provides a deep stretch to the back of the legs.

Improves Flexibility in the Spine: The pose encourages lengthening of the spine, which can help alleviate tension and promote spinal health.

Energizes the Body: An inversion increases blood flow to the brain, which can help boost energy levels and improve focus and concentration.

Tones the Core: Engaging the abdominal muscles to maintain the pose helps to strengthen and tone the core muscles.

Mental Benefits:

Reduces Stress: The inversion aspect of the pose helps improve circulation to the brain, which can reduce stress and mild anxiety.

Enhances Focus: Holding the pose requires concentration and mindfulness, improving overall mental focus and clarity.

Therapeutic Benefits:

Relieves Back Pain: By stretching and strengthening multiple muscle groups, including the spine, Downward-Facing Dog can help alleviate chronic back pain, especially in the lower back.

Improves Digestive Health: The pose encourages blood flow to the digestive tract, which can aid in digestion and help alleviate issues like constipation.

Headache Relief: Increased blood circulation to the brain and relaxation of neck muscles can help reduce headache symptoms.

Sinus Relief: The inverted nature of the pose can also assist in clearing sinuses, which is beneficial for those with sinus conditions.

Caution:

People with high blood pressure, glaucoma, or severe carpal tunnel syndrome should modify this pose or practice with caution. Additionally, those with severe shoulder or wrist injuries may need to avoid this pose until they have healed or found a suitable modification.

Phalakasana (Plank Pose)

Leg Movement: Inhale and extend your left leg back, straightening your torso into a plank position.

Arm Alignment: Ensure your arms are perpendicular to the floor, providing vital support.

Gaze and Spine: Keep your gaze forward and ensure your spine remains straight, forming a straight line from your head to your heels.

Stability and Relaxation: Maintain steadiness in this position while remaining relaxed.

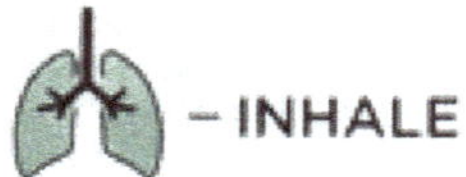

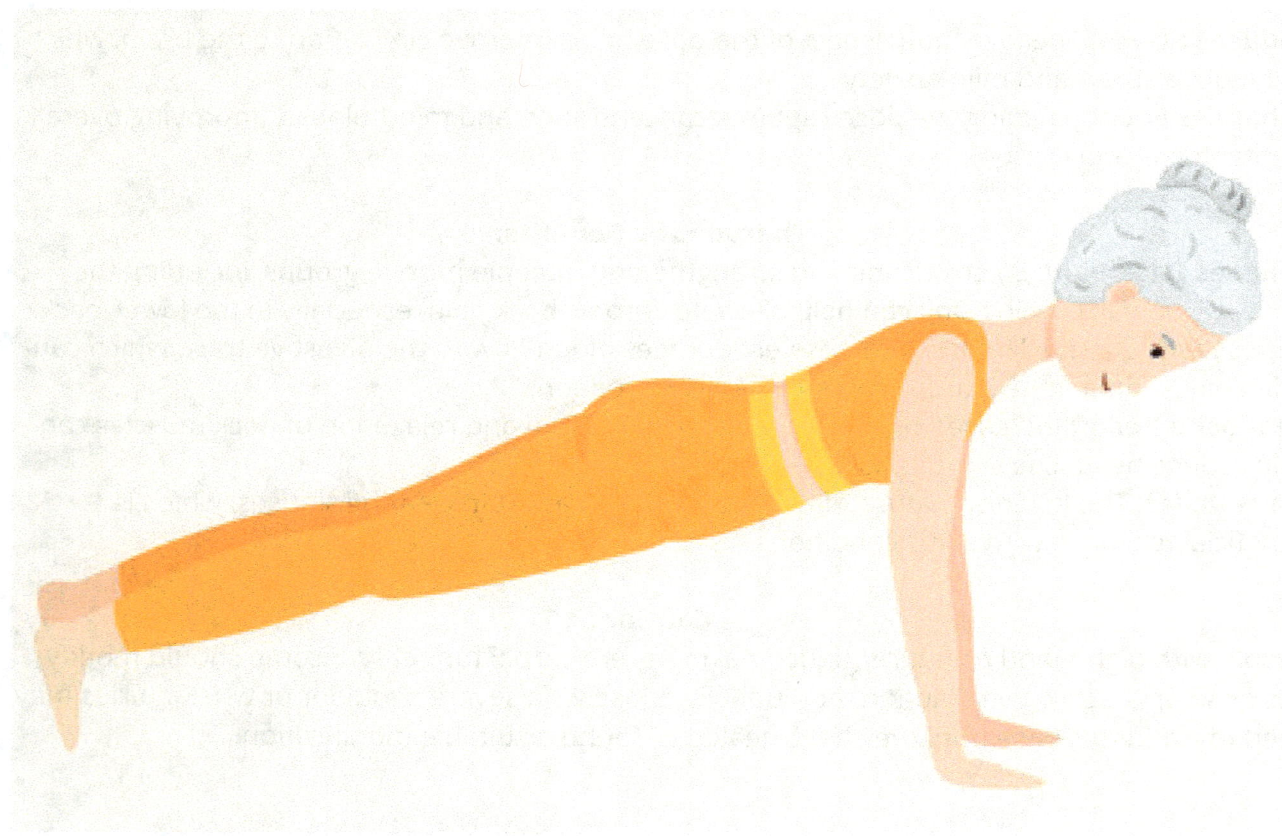

Modifications:

Forearm Plank: Instead of flatting your palms on the mat, lower onto your forearms. This variation reduces stress on the wrists and focuses more on core stabilization. Make sure your elbows are directly under your shoulders to maintain proper alignment.

Knee Plank: Lower your knees to the ground while in the plank position. This reduces the load on your core and makes the pose more accessible. Keep your back straight and core engaged to gain the strength benefits still.

Incline Plank: Elevate your hands using a sturdy piece of furniture or the wall. Place your hands on the edge of a stable chair or against the wall instead of the floor. This decreases the angle of your body relative to the ground, making the pose less intense.

Chair Plank: Sit in a chair and place your hands on the armrests. Press down into the armrests and try to lift your body off the chair seat, keeping your core engaged and your body straight from your head to your knees. This variation significantly reduces strain while engaging the core muscles.

Benefits of Phalakasana:

Strengthens Arms and Back: Phalakasana builds strength in the arms and back, supporting upper body resilience.

Improves Posture: Engaging the core and aligning the body improves posture.

Stretches Shoulders, Chest, and Spine: This pose provides a beneficial stretch to the shoulders, chest, and spine length.

Calms the Mind: Holding the plank position requires concentration and breath control, which can help calm the mind.

Incorporating Phalakasana into your Surya Namaskar practice enhances physical strength and alignment and promotes mental focus and discipline. As a foundational pose, it prepares the body and mind for the complexities of the sequence ahead, embodying the strength and stability that characterize a dedicated yoga practice.

Ashtanga Namaskara Asana (Eight-Limbed Pose)

Following the Plank Pose, transition forward, lowering your chest, knees, and chin to the floor.

Keep your hips slightly elevated, not touching the ground, ensuring that eight parts of the body (two hands, two feet, two knees, chest, and chin) touch the floor.

Find stability and relaxation in this pose, gently engaging your core and leg muscles to maintain the position.

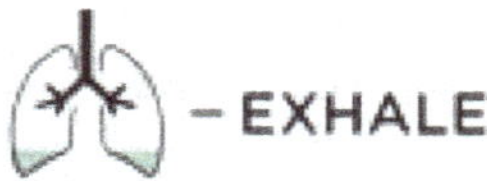

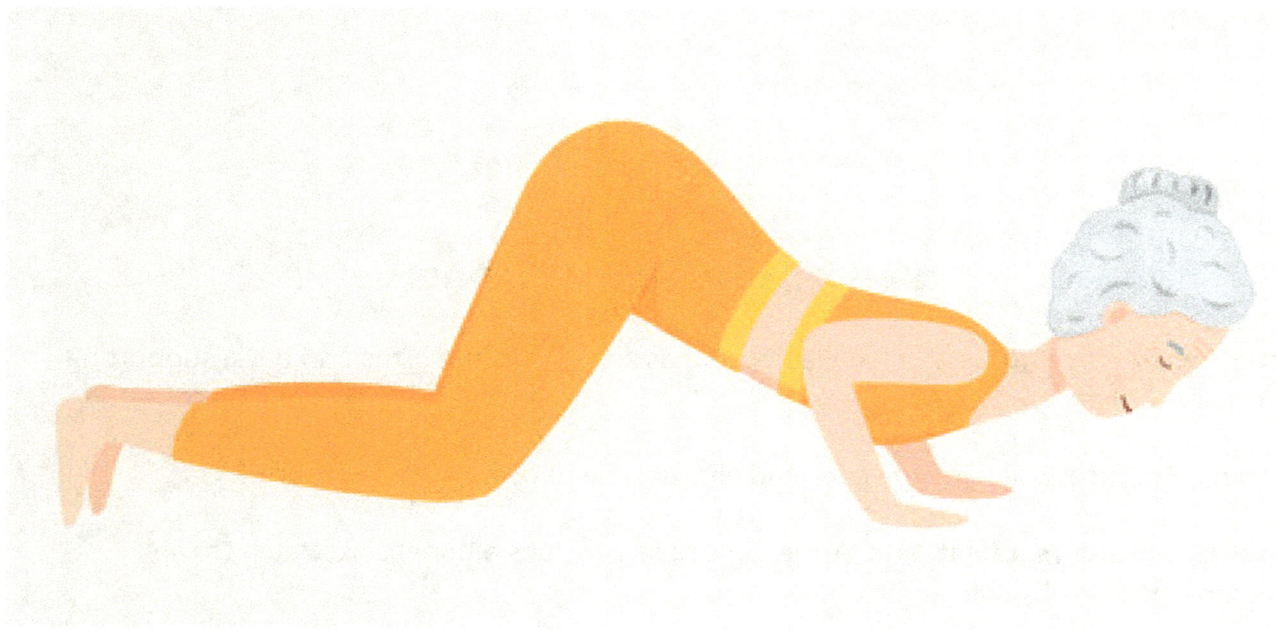

Modifications for Seniors - Eight-Limbed Pose

Cushions or Blankets: Place cushions or folded blankets under the chest and thighs to lessen the impact and provide support, reducing the strain on your body.

Yoga Blocks: Use yoga blocks under the hands to help support your weight, reducing pressure on your wrists and shoulders.

Tabletop Chest and Chin Touch:
Start in a tabletop position with your knees and hands on the mat.
Lower the chest and chin to the mat, keeping the hips aligned over the knees. This variation reduces the intensity and focuses on gentle stretching and strengthening without the total body weight bearing down.

Standing Variation:
Use a wall for support. Stand facing the wall and lean forward until your chest and chin gently touch the wall, keeping the rest of the body upright. This simulates the pose without getting down on the floor.

Physical and mental benefits of Eight-Limbed Pose

Physical Benefits:

Strengthens Muscles: Ashtanga Namaskara strengthens the arms, shoulders, and back muscles as you support your body weight with your hands and feet. It also engages the core muscles, enhancing core stability and strength.

Improves Flexibility: The pose helps increase flexibility in the back and hips as the body stretches back and forth between the supportive points.

Enhances Body Awareness: Balancing on eight points requires concentration and body awareness, helping to improve proprioception (the sense of the relative position of body parts).

Mental Benefits:

Develops Focus and Concentration: Maintaining the pose and balancing the body weight on multiple points requires and thus improves focus and concentration.

Reduces Stress and Anxiety: The pose is often practiced as part of a sequence that promotes relaxation and stress relief, reducing overall anxiety levels.

Promotes Discipline and Patience: Mastering this pose and its integration into flowing sequences like the Sun Salutation requires practice, discipline, and patience.

Additional Benefits:

Promotes Humility and Grounding: Ashtanga Namaskara is a posture that brings you close to the earth, promoting feelings of humility and grounding.

Prepares for More Advanced Poses: Practicing this pose can prepare the body for more advanced poses that require strength, balance, and flexibility.
This pose is beneficial in sequences where gradual warming up of the body is required, making it ideal for beginning or deepening a yoga practice. However, due to its complexity and the needed strength, it is essential to perform it properly to avoid strain, especially in the wrists and lower back.

Bhujangasana (Cobra Pose)

Inhale and slide forward, raising your chest off the ground while looking up towards the ceiling.

Ensure your elbows are bent and shoulders away from your ears, creating an arch in your back from the navel upward, legs together.

For a deeper stretch, you may push your chest forward as you inhale; gently lower your abdomen towards the floor as you exhale, avoiding overstretching.

Stabilize and relax in the pose before moving on.

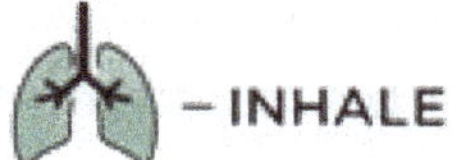

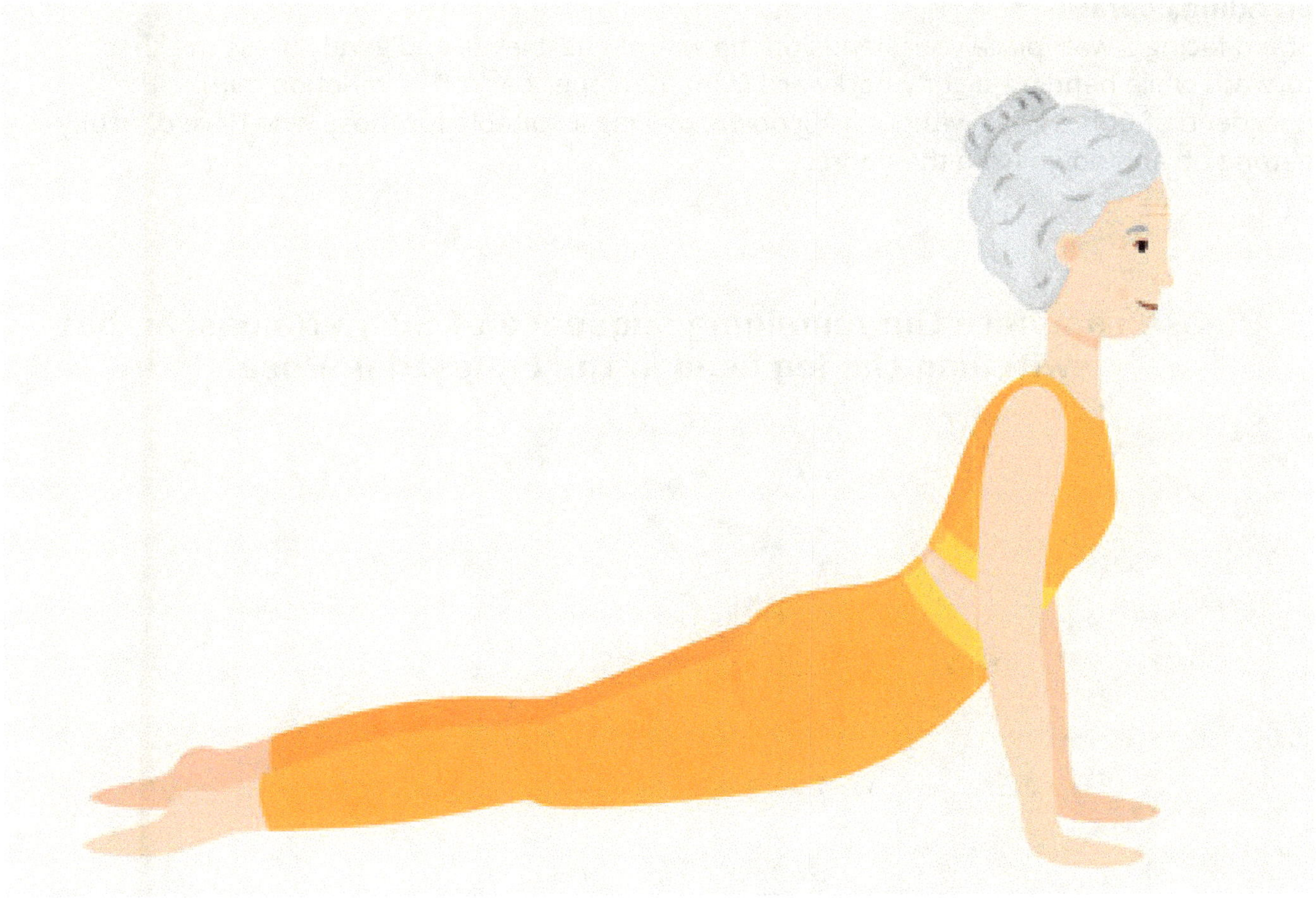

Modifications for Seniors

Gentle Lift:
Instead of lifting high, seniors can perform a very gentle lift, raising the chest just a few inches off the ground. This reduces the strain on the lower back and still helps to strengthen the spine.

Using Elbows for Support:
Place the forearms on the ground with elbows directly under the shoulders, creating a "Sphinx Pose." This modification still opens the chest and strengthens the spine, reducing the backbend intensity.

Hands Positioned Further Forward:
Move the hands forward, away from the shoulders, to create a less intense backbend. This can help alleviate pressure on the lower back while engaging the muscles needed for the pose.

Use Props for Support:
Place a rolled towel or a small cushion under the hips to provide extra support and reduce pressure on the lower back. This can help ease discomfort and make the pose more accessible.

Standing Cobra:
Stand facing a wall, place your hands on the wall at chest level, and gently press the chest forward while bending slightly backward from the upper back. This variation mimics the backbend of Cobra Pose without lying down, making it suitable for those who have difficulty getting up and down from the floor.

Please complete the remaining sequence of Surya Namaskar, but switching the leg used in the Equestrian Pose.

Benefits

Physical Benefits:

Strengthens the Spine: Regular practice of Bhujangasana helps strengthen the muscles around the spine, improving flexibility and potentially reducing the symptoms of chronic back pain.

Opens the Chest and Shoulders: This pose encourages the opening of the chest, which helps improve lung capacity and counteract the forward slump often observed in older adults. It also helps relieve stiffness around the shoulders and upper back.

Stimulates Abdominal Organs: The gentle pressure on the abdomen during Bhujangasana helps stimulate abdominal organs, aiding in better digestion and helping relieve constipation.

Enhances Posture: By strengthening the spine and opening the chest, Cobra Pose promotes better alignment and posture, which is crucial for overall health and mobility in seniors.

Mental Benefits:

Reduces Stress: The pose has a calming effect on the nervous system, which can help reduce anxiety and elevate mood, promoting a general sense of well-being.

Increases Energy and Vitality: This gentle backbend stimulates the body and can increase energy levels, helping to overcome feelings of lethargy.

Therapeutic Benefits:

Relieves Symptoms of Sciatica: Cobra Pose can help alleviate mild sciatica pain by stretching and strengthening the spine.

May Help in Managing Respiratory Conditions: The chest opening improves breathing capacity, benefiting seniors with asthma or chronic bronchitis.

Caution:

While Bhujangasana is generally safe, it should be approached with caution, especially by those with severe spinal disorders, recent abdominal surgeries, or hernias. Always begin with a gentle version of the pose, and avoid overextending the back, which can lead to strain or injury. A folded towel or blanket under the hips can provide additional support and comfort.

Deep Relaxation: Savasana

Each practice should conclude with Savasana, which is essential for integrating the benefits of the session.

Savasana, often called the Corpse Pose, holds unparalleled significance in yoga, transcending its apparent simplicity. This concluding pose of a yoga sequence is a gateway to profound inner tranquility, facilitating a deep connection with the inner self.

The Essence of Savasana

Profound Relaxation: Savasana is the key to unlocking a state of comprehensive relaxation, encompassing both the physical and mental dimensions. Complete stillness and focused breath awareness allow for unwinding accumulated stress, fostering a rejuvenating effect.

Alleviation of Stress:

Activating the body's parasympathetic nervous system, Savasana aids in diminishing stress, lowering the heart rate, reducing blood pressure, and instilling a sense of serenity.

Augmented Self-awareness:

The tranquil state induced by Savasana offers an enhanced sense of mindfulness and self-reflection. It nurtures a space where the mind can observe without judgment, cultivating a more profound understanding of being.

Consolidation of Benefits:

This pose is crucial for the body to internalize and integrate the physical and subtle energies mobilized through the preceding asanas. It's akin to allowing the body to 'absorb' the essence of the practice.

Emotional Equilibrium:

Savasana provides a rare sanctuary of stillness, facilitating the release of emotional tension and fostering emotional steadiness and resilience.

Gateway to Meditation:

The profound relaxation and mental clarity achieved in Savasana lay the groundwork for more profound meditative practices, easing the transition into meditation.

Embracing the Depth of Savasana:

Savasana's transformative power is unveiled through intentional practice and surrender. It demands a conscious release of control over breath, body, and thoughts, inviting a state of complete surrender.

Corpse Pose (Savasana) - Detailed Instruction:
Positioning:

Start by lying on your back on a yoga mat or a comfortable surface, ensuring your spine is straight and your legs are extended. Allow your feet to fall naturally to the sides. If lying flat causes discomfort in your lower back, consider sliding a bolster or rolled blanket under your knees for support.

Place your arms alongside your body but slightly separated from your torso. Turn your palms to face upwards, signaling your body to open up and relax fully. Ensure your shoulder blades are evenly spread and lightly tucked under to open the chest.

Gently close your eyes to signal your body that it's time to wind down. Make any adjustments you need to feel completely comfortable and symmetrical. The idea is to eliminate physical distractions that might prevent you from fully relaxing.

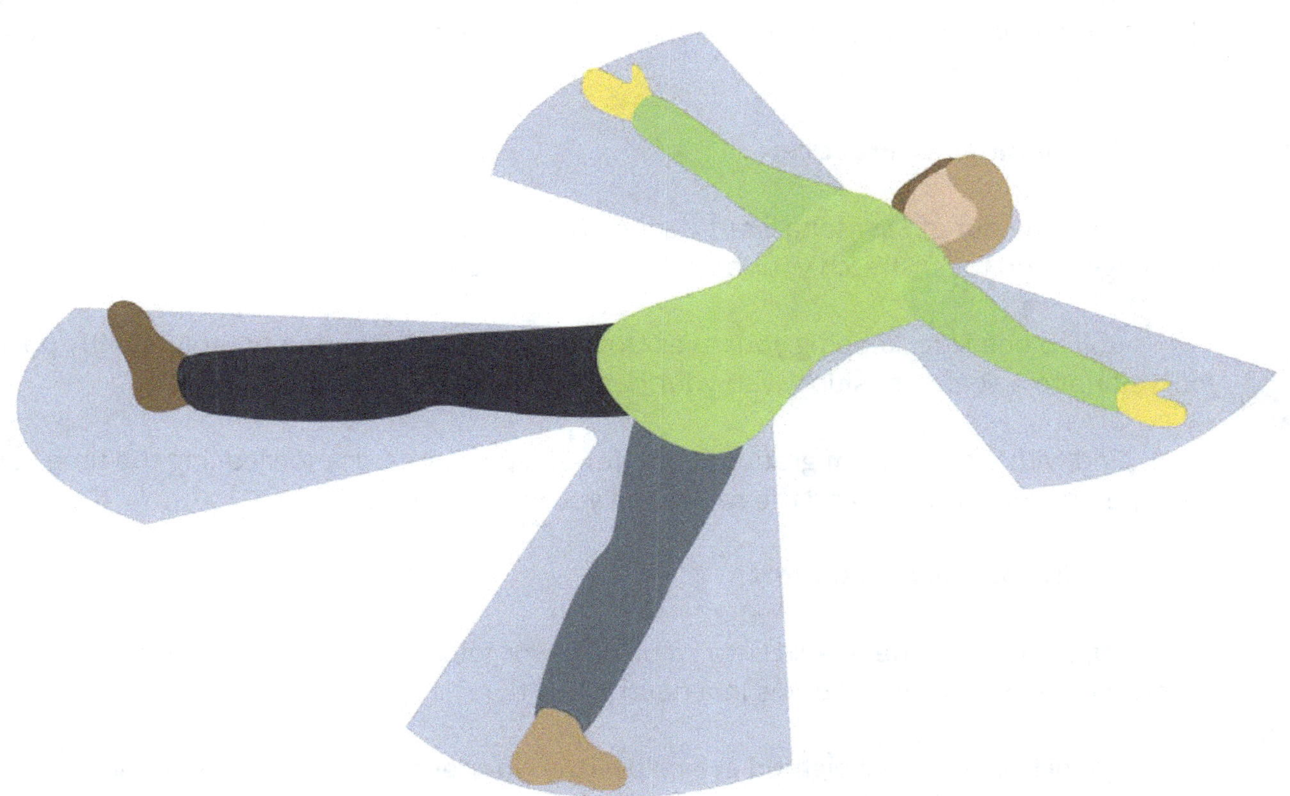

Entering Relaxation:

Take a few deep breaths, inhaling through the nose and exhaling through the mouth. With each exhale, imagine releasing any tension in your body.

Progressive muscle relaxation: Starting at the crown of your head and moving down to your toes, consciously relax each part of your body. Spend a few breaths on each area, mentally releasing any tension.

Mindfulness and letting go: Turn your attention to your breath. Notice the natural rhythm of your inhalations and exhalations without trying to change anything. If your mind wanders, gently acknowledge the thought and bring your attention back to your breath.

Techniques for Deep Relaxation:

Visualization: Imagine a wave of relaxation slowly moving through your body, starting at your head and flowing down to your toes. With each wave, your body becomes lighter and more relaxed.

Counting breaths: Silently count your breaths backward from 100 to 1. If you lose track, start again. This technique can help keep your mind focused and prevent it from wandering.

Mantra repetition: Choose a calming word or phrase, such as "peace" or "I am relaxed." Silently repeat your mantra with each inhale and exhale, allowing the repetition to anchor your mind in the present moment.

Concluding the Practice:

To come out of Savasana, start deepening your breath, bringing gentle movement back to your fingers and toes. Stretch your arms overhead for a full-body stretch.

Roll to one side, keeping your eyes closed, and rest there momentarily. Gently push yourself up to a seated position with your hands.

End with a moment of gratitude or a few deep breaths, acknowledging the time you've dedicated to your practice and the relaxation you've cultivated.

Modifications for Comfort:

Support under the head: Use a small pillow or folded blanket under your head if it tilts back too far, ensuring your neck is in a neutral position.

Eye pillow: Place a weighted eye pillow over your eyes to block out light and help deepen your relaxation.

Covering: Use a light blanket to cover your body. This will keep you warm as your body temperature drops and provide security and comfort.

Savasana is a crucial component of yoga, offering deep relaxation and integrating the benefits of your physical practice. By permitting yourself to rest fully, you allow the body to assimilate the work done during the session, leading to a refreshed and rejuvenated state.

Closing: Thanksgiving and Reflection
Gently Awaken: Slowly bring movement back to your body by wiggling your fingers and toes. Roll to one side and gradually rise to a seated position.
Return to Prayer Pose: Bring your palms together in front of your heart, reflecting on your practice and the fulfillment of your Sankalpa.
Express Gratitude: Silently or aloud, express thanks for your practice, your body's capabilities, and the peace and insight gained.

Close Your Practice: With a final inhalation, lift your palms slightly above your head, then exhale and lower your hands back to your heart, sealing in the benefits of your practice.

Namaste holds even more profound significance. It marks the culmination of a practice, sealing the shared experience of unity, peace, and harmony. It's an expression of gratitude from teacher to student and from student back to the teacher, acknowledging the journey they've embarked on together. Namaste serves as a bridge, connecting the physical to the spiritual, the individual to the collective, grounding the practice in humility and reverence.

Remember, this practice is a journey, not a destination. Each day and practice are opportunities to explore deeper aspects of yourself and connect with the vast expanse of your inner world.

Day 1
Root Chakra (MULADHARA):
The foundation of the chakra system, located at the base of the spine, represents our sense of security, survival, and belonging.
It's element is Earth

Signs of a Balanced :
A strong sense of grounding and connection to the Earth
Feelings of security and stability
Confidence in facing life's challenges
A healthy physical existence

Signs of an Imbalance:
Excessive fear and anxiety about security and survival
Feeling disconnected or alienated from one's surroundings
Physical issues related to the lower body, such as lower back pain or leg discomfort
Financial difficulties or an unhealthy focus on material possessions

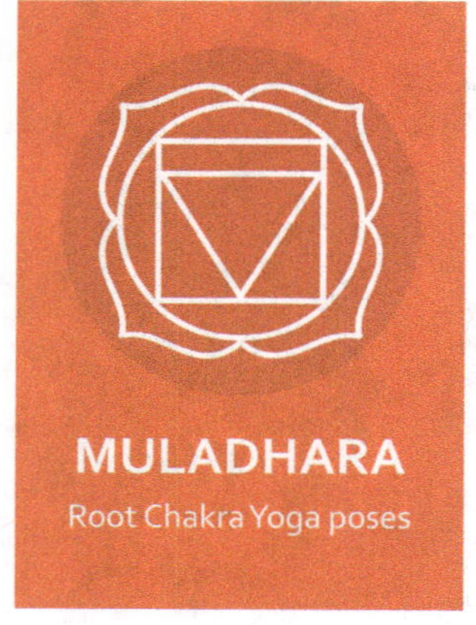

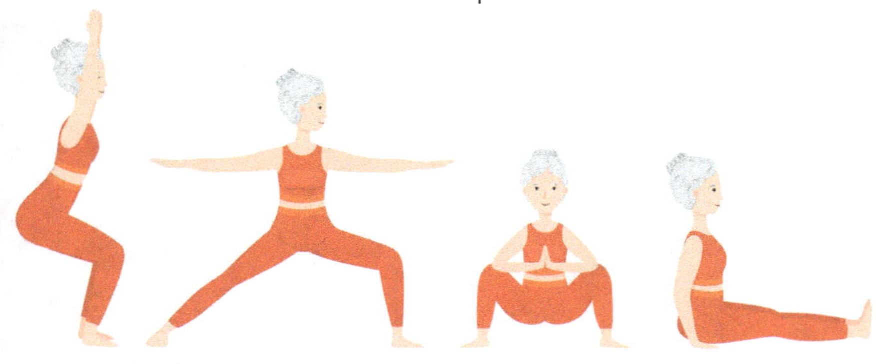

Use affirmations such as
"I am grounded and secure,"
"I trust in the abundance of life,"
"I have everything I need for a fulfilling life."

Pranayama:
Close your eyes and take several deep, slow breaths. Inhale through your nose and exhale through your mouth. Let your breathing become slow and steady.

Meditation:
Imagine a bright red glowing light at the base of your spine. Visualize this red light expanding and growing stronger with each breath. This light represents the energy of the root chakra.

The Chair Pose (Utkatasana)

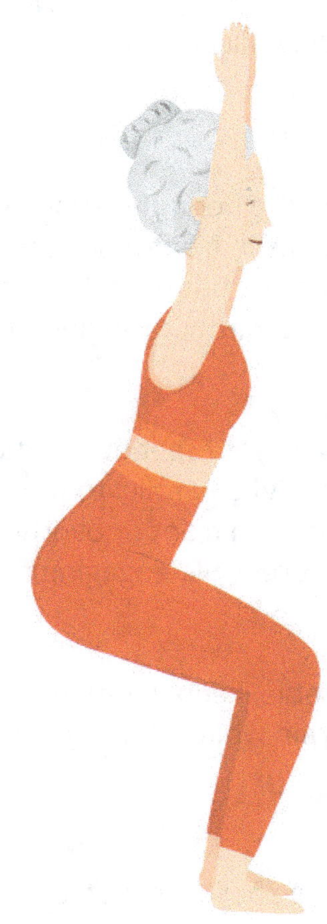

Start: In Mountain Pose, stand with feet hip-width or together. Feel grounded.

Bend Knees: Exhale, bend your knees like sitting back in a chair, thighs aiming parallel to the floor. Ensure knees don't pass toes.

Raise Arms: Inhale and lift arms overhead, parallel, with palms facing in.

Shoulders relaxed.

Core Engagement: Draw the navel to the spine and tuck the tailbone slightly.

Stability Focus: Weight back into heels, visualize roots extending from feet into the earth.

Hold: Maintain for 5-10 breaths, feeling the earth's support.

Release: Inhale and straighten your legs and arms up. Exhale, lower arms, returning to Mountain Pose.

Stand behind a chair and hold onto the back for support. Lower into a partial squat, keeping the knees in line with the feet and not extending past the toes. This helps maintain balance and reduces the load on the legs.

Seated Chair Pose:
Sit on the edge of a chair with your feet on the floor and spaced together. Lean slightly forward, keeping your back straight, and lift your arms in front of you, parallel to the floor. Engage your core and thighs as if you are about to stand up, but hold the position to create muscle tension. This version strengthens the thighs and core without the need for standing.

Wall-Supported Chair Pose:
Stand with your back against a wall and walk your feet out a little while sliding your back down the wall into a seated position. Keep your thighs parallel to the floor, or as close as possible, and your knees over your ankles. Raise your arms in front or overhead as comfort allows. This modification reduces knee and back pressure while engaging the leg muscles.

Hand Position Variations:
If raising the arms overhead is uncomfortable, keep your hands together at your chest in prayer or on your hips. This reduces shoulder strain while allowing you to focus on strengthening your legs and core.

Reduced Squat Depth:
Instead of lowering down deeply, perform a shallow squat, only bending the knees slightly. This is easier on the knees and helps build strength in the legs and hips.

Key benefits of practicing Chair Pose:

Physical Benefits:
Strengthens the Lower Body: Chair Pose deeply works the muscles of the thighs and calves, strengthening the quadriceps, hamstrings, and ankles. It also engages the glutes, making it a comprehensive lower-body workout.
Tones the Core: As you hold the pose, your core muscles must engage to maintain balance and stability, helping to strengthen and tone the abdominal muscles.
Improves Posture: The pose requires a straight spine and engaged torso, which helps improve overall posture and spine health. Regular practice can also help alleviate some forms of back pain by strengthening the supportive muscles of the back.
Increases Stamina and Heat in the Body: Holding the Chair Pose builds heat and can increase stamina. It's an energizing pose that can help invigorate the entire body.

Mental Benefits:
Enhances Focus and Determination: Maintaining the pose requires concentration and mental endurance, which can improve overall mental focus and determination.
Relieves Stress: Although physically demanding, the intense focus required can help divert attention from daily stressors, providing a mental break.
Therapeutic Benefits:
Stimulates the Diaphragm and Heart: The upright, engaged position of the torso stimulates the heart and diaphragm, improving blood circulation and aiding in respiratory functions.
Balances Metabolism: The chair pose can help regulate and balance metabolism by stimulating the digestive organs through its slight bend and twist in the torso.

Caution:
Chair Pose can be intense on the knees and the lower back. Those with chronic knee pain, arthritis, or lower back issues should approach this pose cautiously or seek modifications, such as not bending as profoundly, to make it more accessible.

Overall, the Chair Pose is a robust posture that benefits the mind and body, providing both physical strengthening and mental rejuvenation.

Warrior I (Virabhadrasana I&II)

Start in Mountain Pose: Stand tall, feet together.

Step Feet Apart: Approximately 4 to 5 feet.

Raise Arms: Extend your arms to the sides at shoulder height, palms down.

Turn Left Foot Out: Rotate your left foot 90 degrees and your right foot slightly.

Bend Left Knee: Bend your left knee over the ankle and thigh parallel to the floor.

Gaze Over Left Hand: Turn your head to look over your left hand.

Hold and Breathe: Stay for five breaths, then switch sides.

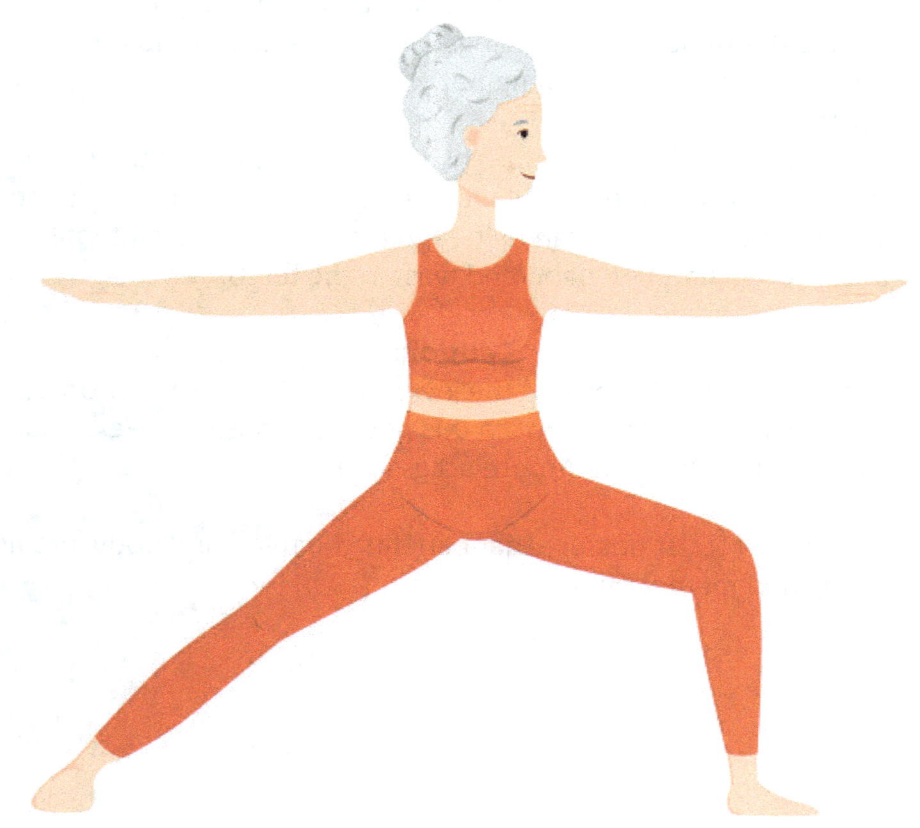

Use a Chair for Support:
Position a chair before you and step your front foot between the chair legs. Keep your back foot at a comfortable angle with the heel down or slightly lifted, depending on what feels best. Hold the back of the chair with one or both hands for balance as you bend the front knee.
For a deeper pose, you can place the back foot on the ground, aligning the heel with the front heel or slightly wider for more stability.

Wall Support:
Stand with your back near a wall for added balance and security. Use the wall to steady yourself with one hand while you practice stepping one foot forward and bending the knee, keeping the other hand raised if possible.

Shorten the Stance:
Decrease the distance between your feet. A shorter stance reduces the intensity of the stretch in the legs and makes it easier to maintain balance.

Reduce Arm Strain:
Instead of raising the arms overhead, which can be challenging for those with shoulder issues, place your hands on your hips or keep them in a prayer position at your chest. You can also extend them parallel to the floor to reduce shoulder strain.

Adjust Back Foot Position:
Instead of turning the back foot out 45 degrees, which can be challenging on the hips and balance, allow the foot to point more towards the front of the mat or keep it parallel to the short edge of the mat. This can be more comfortable and help maintain hip alignment.

Key benefits of practicing Warrior I:

Physical Benefits:

Strengthens the Lower Body: Warrior I works extensively on the leg muscles, strengthening the quadriceps, hamstrings, and calves. It also increases the flexibility in the hips and helps stabilize the knees and ankles.

Tones the Upper Body: The arms are held up and back, strengthening the shoulders, arms, and back muscles. It also helps improve the flexibility and strength of the spine.

Improves Core Stability: Holding the pose requires and builds core strength, essential for overall body balance and stability.

Enhances Respiratory Capacity: The upward stretch of the arms and the opening of the chest help to expand the lungs, which increases breathing capacity and improves overall respiratory function.

Mental Benefits:

Increases Focus and Concentration: The pose requires a balance of strength and grace, which demands concentration and presence of mind, thus enhancing mental clarity.

Boosts Energy and Stamina: Warrior I is energizing, helping to reduce fatigue and boost physical and mental stamina.

Therapeutic Benefits:

Alleviates Sciatica and Back Pain: Regular practice can help relieve back pain and sciatica symptoms by strengthening and stretching the spine and lower back muscles.

Improves Circulation: The active nature of the pose stimulates blood flow throughout the body, which can help improve heart function and overall circulation.

Additional Benefits:

Encourages Good Alignment and Posture: The pose promotes the alignment of the hips and shoulders, which can correct postural imbalances and alleviate issues stemming from poor posture.

Reduces Stress and Calms the Mind: By focusing on the pose and maintaining steady, deep breaths, Warrior I can help reduce stress and promote a calm, clear mind.

Caution:

People with severe hip, knee, or shoulder problems should approach Warrior I with caution or avoid it altogether. Modifications can accommodate various conditions, such as adjusting the leg distance or limiting the arm raise to reduce strain.

Overall, Warrior I is a comprehensive pose that enhances physical and mental health, promoting strength, flexibility, and resilience.

Squat Pose (Malasana)

Start Position: Stand with feet about mat-width apart, toes slightly turned out.

Lower Down: Exhale and squat down, keeping your heels on the floor if possible. If not, support heels on a folded mat or blanket.

Elbows Inside Knees: Bring your elbows to the inside of your knees, palms together in prayer position, and gently press your elbows against your knees.

Chest Lifted: Keep your spine straight and chest lifted.

Hold: Breathe deeply in this pose for 30 seconds to a minute.

Release: To come out, exhale, and straighten your legs, returning to a standing position.

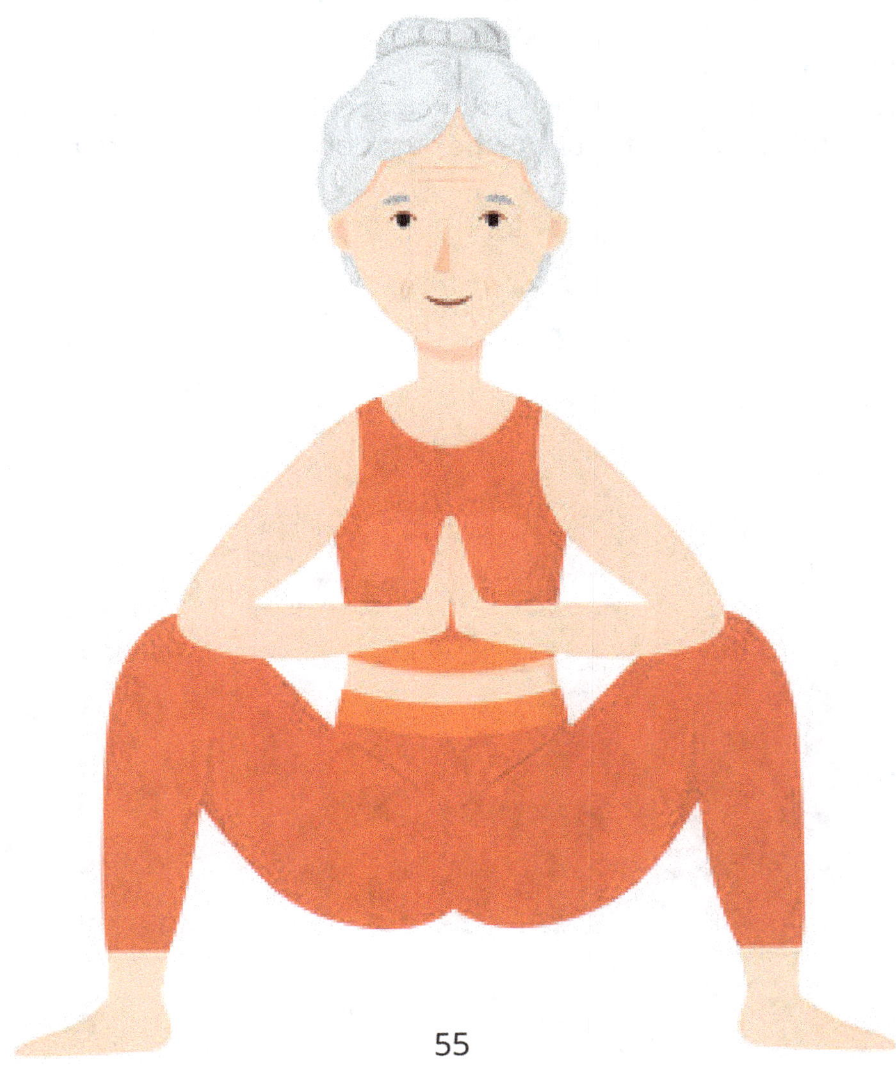

Use Props for Support:
If the heels don't comfortably reach the floor, place a yoga block or a folded blanket under them. This provides stability and can help maintain balance.
Sit on a yoga block or a cushion to reduce the depth of the squat, which lessens the strain on the knees and hips.

Chair Malasana:
Perform the pose while seated at the edge of a chair. Separate your thighs slightly wider than hip-width, with feet flat on the floor. Lean forward gently with a straight back, pressing your elbows against your inner knees to mimic Malasana's action. This variation provides the hip-opening benefits without the balance and mobility demands of the full squat.

Wall Support:
Stand with your back against a wall to perform Malasana. Slide down into a squat while using the wall for back support. This helps maintain balance and reduces the load on the legs.

Hold Onto Something Stable:
You can use a sturdy piece of furniture or a countertop to hold onto while squatting down. This helps with balance and allows you to control the depth of the squat according to your comfort level.

Key benefits of incorporating Malasana

Physical Benefits:

Enhances Hip Flexibility: Malasana profoundly opens the hips, increasing flexibility and mobility in the hip joints, which can benefit overall movement and posture.
Strengthens the Lower Body: The pose strengthens the ankles, legs, and lower back, as the lower limbs support the body's weight.
Tones the Abdomen: Engaging the core throughout the pose helps to tone the abdominal muscles, contributing to better core stability.
Improves Balance and Posture: Practicing Malasana challenges and improves balance, enhancing overall posture and coordination.

Mental Benefits:

Promotes Calmness: Holding the pose requires focus and deep breathing, which can help calm the mind and reduce stress and anxiety.
Encourages Mindfulness: The intense focus required in maintaining balance and alignment in this pose helps foster a state of mindfulness, keeping you present in the moment.

Therapeutic Benefits:

Aids in Digestion: The squatting position can help facilitate bowel movements and alleviate bloating by compressing the abdomen and stimulating the digestive organs.
Relieves Lower Back Pain: Malasana can help alleviate tension and pain in the lower back by stretching the back and strengthening the core and lower back muscles.
Improves Circulation in the Legs: The pose promotes blood flow to the pelvis and lower extremities, which can help reduce swelling and fatigue in the legs.

"Dandasana," or Staff Pose.

Starting Position:
Sit on a yoga mat or a folded blanket for extra cushioning. This elevation can help if you have tight hamstrings or lower back issues.

Leg Position:
Extend your legs straight out in front of you. Keep your feet together or slightly apart, whichever feels more comfortable.

If your hamstrings are tight, consider placing a rolled towel or a small bolster under your knees for support. This modification helps reduce strain on your lower back.

Upper Body Alignment:
Sit up straight. Imagine a string pulling your head towards the ceiling, elongating your spine. Place your palms flat on the mat beside your hips to support your posture. If this is uncomfortable, you can place your hands slightly behind you with fingers pointing away or towards your body.

Engage Your Core:
Gently engage your abdominal muscles to support your spine. Keep your chest open and shoulders relaxed.

Foot and Leg Activation:
Flex your feet to engage the muscles in your legs. Press your heels away from you and pull your toes towards your body.

Breath:
Breathe deeply and evenly, maintaining a relaxed face and jaw. Focus on maintaining a steady and slow breath, which aids in maintaining balance and focus in the pose.

Hold and Release:
Hold the pose for 30 seconds to 1 minute, or as long as comfortable. To release, relax your legs and sit comfortably in a relaxed position.

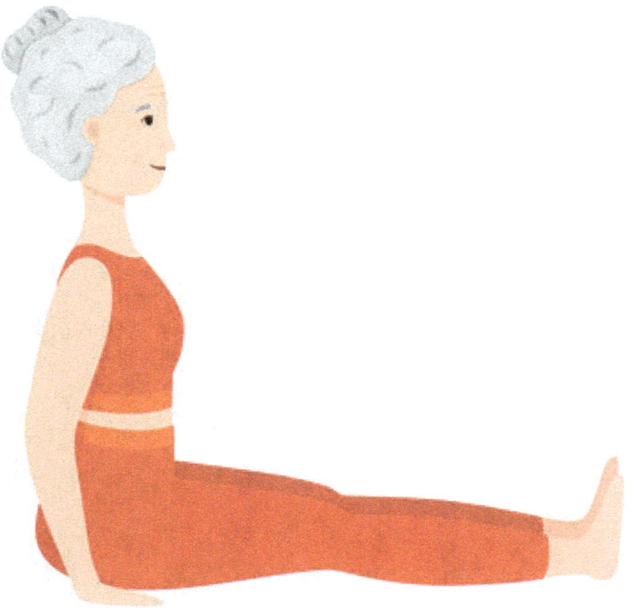

Key benefits of practicing Dandasana

Physical Benefits:

Strengthens Core Muscles: Dandasana requires you to engage your abdominal muscles to maintain an upright posture, which helps strengthen the core and improve posture and balance.

Improves Posture: Sitting upright with a straight back trains the back and shoulder muscles, which are essential for good posture. Regular practice of Dandasana can help correct poor posture habits.

Stretches the Hamstrings: The pose involves keeping the legs straight out in front, which stretches the hamstrings and can help alleviate tightness in the back of the legs.

Enhances Flexibility in the Shoulders and Chest: Dandasana helps improve flexibility and mobility in the shoulders and chest by keeping the arms active and the chest open.

Mental Benefits:

Develop Focus and Concentration: The pose requires mental focus to maintain the correct posture, which can help improve overall concentration and mindfulness.

Calms the Mind: The simplicity and static nature of the pose provide a grounding effect, which can help calm the mind, reducing stress and anxiety.

Therapeutic Benefits:

Aids Digestion: The upright posture in Dandasana helps stimulate the abdominal organs, including the digestive system, which can improve digestion and alleviate issues like constipation.

Relieves Back Conditions: By strengthening the core and the muscles along the spine, Dandasana can help relieve conditions associated with weak back muscles and poor posture.

Caution:

While Dandasana is generally safe, individuals with lower back problems should approach this pose cautiously. A folded blanket or cushion under the hips can help maintain proper alignment and reduce strain on the lower back.

Overall, Dandasana offers essential benefits that are fundamental to a balanced yoga practice. It enhances physical stability, posture, and mental clarity. Both beginners and advanced practitioners can integrate this pose into their routines to support a wide range of physical and mental health goals.

Day 2

Sacral Chakra (Svadhishthana):
The Sacral Chakra, located in the lower abdomen, is the center of creativity, emotional balance, and sexuality.
Its element is Water.

Indicators of a Balanced:
Emotional stability and the ability to express emotions freely
Healthy interpersonal relationships and intimacy
Creativity and inspiration
A joyful outlook on life

Signs of Imbalance:
Emotional over-sensitivity or numbness
Fear of pleasure or unhealthy indulgence in pleasure
Creative blocks
Difficulties in relationships and expressing sexuality healthily

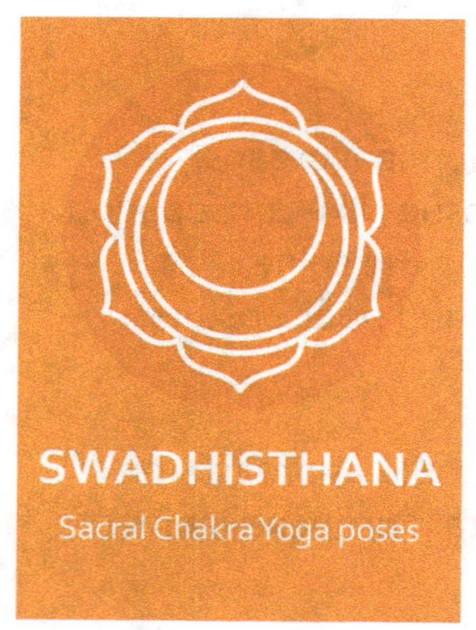

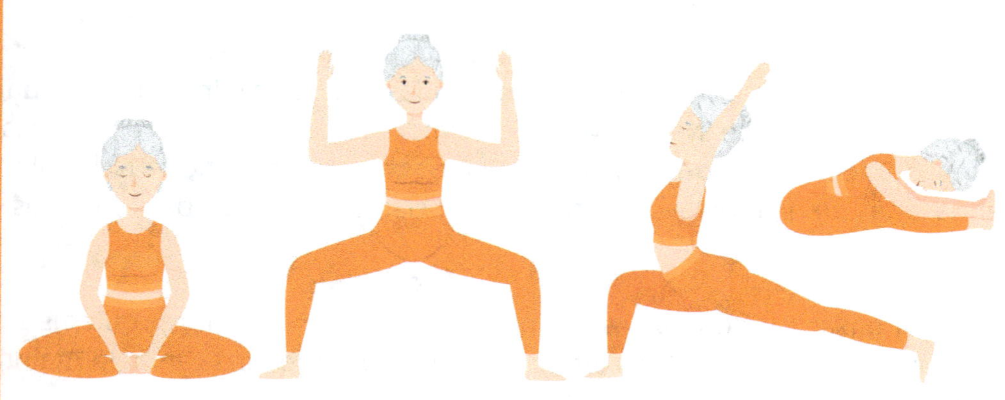

Use affirmations such as
"I deserve happiness, love, and fulfillment"
"I am in touch with my feelings and I honor my emotional needs."
to reinforce the pose's energetic intentions.

Pranayama:
Breathing practices that encourage the flow of prana (life energy) through the sacral region, including Kapalabhati (Skull Shining Breath) and Nadi Shodhana (Alternate Nostril Breathing)

Meditation:
As you settle into your breath, begin to visualize an orange glow at your sacral chakra, located two inches below your navel. Imagine this orange light growing brighter and warmer with each breath.

Goddess Pose (Utkata Konasana)

Start Position: Stand with your feet wider than hip-distance apart, turning your toes to about 45 degrees.

Bend Knees: Exhale as you bend your knees over your toes, lowering your hips into a squat. Aim to bring your thighs parallel to the ground, but adjust depth according to comfort.

Arm Position: Raise your arms to shoulder height, bending the elbows to form a 90-degree angle, palms facing forward or touching in prayer at your heart.

Engage Core: Keep your core engaged, tailbone tucked slightly, and chest lifted.

Hold and Breathe: Maintain the pose for 30 seconds to a minute, focusing on deep, steady breaths.

To Release: Straighten your legs and lower your arms, returning to standing.

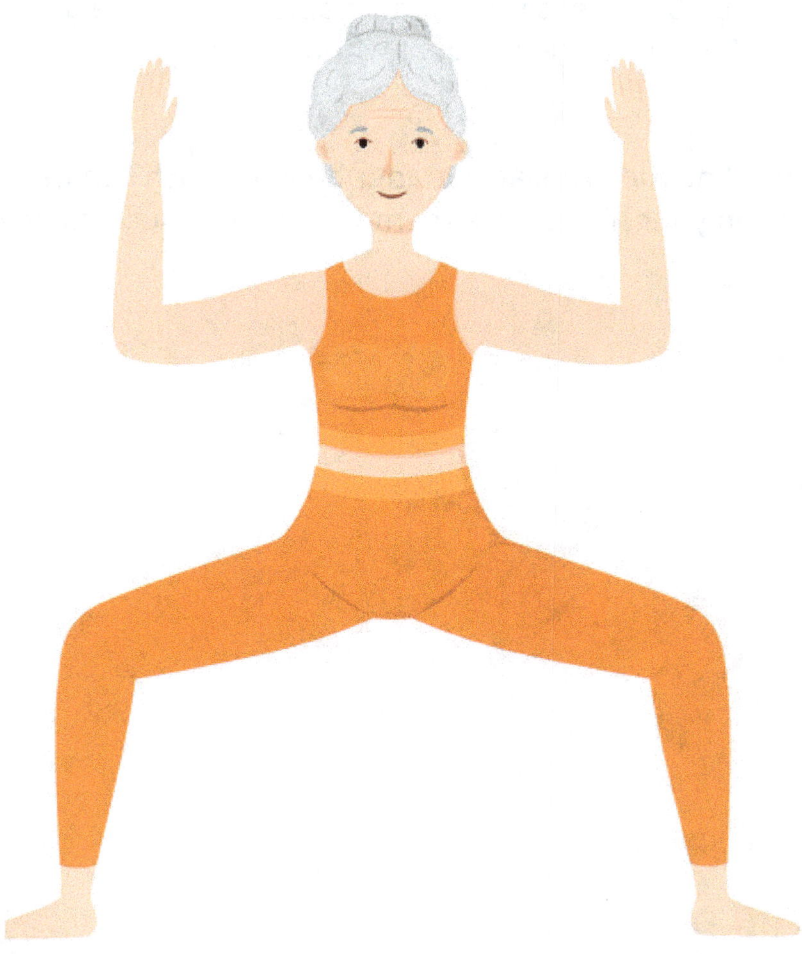

Modifications for Seniors

Chair Support:

A sturdy chair is your best friend in this pose. Position it in front of you and grip the back with both hands. This not only ensures balance but also allows you to focus on engaging your legs and hips, making it an ideal starting point for beginners.

Shallow Bend:

Instead of bending deeply into the squat, perform a shallower knee bend. This reduces the strain on the knees and hips while providing a good stretch and strengthening the thighs.

Wall Support:

Stand with your back near a wall and slide down into a squat as comfortably as possible. The wall supports your back, helping you maintain balance and alignment.

Foot Position:

If turning the feet to 45 degrees is uncomfortable, reduce the angle slightly. Keep your feet at a comfortable angle to squat without pain.

Hand Position:

Rather than extending the arms at shoulder height, which can be strenuous, please keep your hands on your hips or use them for support (such as holding onto a chair or wall).

Key benefits of practicing Goddess Pose

Physical Benefits:

Strengthens the Lower Body: Goddess Pose intensely works the muscles of the thighs, calves, and glutes. It helps build strength and stamina in the legs.

Opens the Hips and Chest: The wide stance and outward rotation of the hips help to increase hip flexibility. Simultaneously, the pose encourages an open, expansive chest, which stretches the chest muscles and strengthens the upper back.

Improves Core Stability: Maintaining balance and alignment in this pose requires a solid and engaged core, which improves overall stability and supports spinal health.

Enhances Circulation: The dynamic nature of the pose stimulates blood flow throughout the body, energizing the systems and improving overall circulatory health.

Mental Benefits:

Boosts Confidence and Empowerment: The pose's powerful stance and energetic openness can help boost confidence and create a sense of empowerment and strength.

Reduces Stress: Goddess Pose can help reduce stress and anxiety by focusing on deep breathing and maintaining a robust and stable posture.

Therapeutic Benefits:

Alleviates Symptoms of Menopause: The pose helps to stimulate the reproductive organs and can be beneficial in alleviating some of the symptoms associated with menopause.

Supports Pelvic Floor Health: The squatting action and engagement required in Goddess Pose help tone and strengthen the pelvic floor muscles, which is beneficial for sexual health and urinary function.

Additional Benefits:

Promotes Balance and Coordination: Holding this pose and maintaining balance helps improve physical coordination and awareness.

Energizing: Goddess Pose can be particularly invigorating, making it a great addition to a morning yoga routine or any time you need an energy boost.

Caution:

While Goddess Pose is generally safe for most individuals, those with hip, knee, or ankle issues should approach this pose cautiously or seek modifications. For example, adjusting the depth of the squat or the distance between the feet can help accommodate individual needs and limitations.

Goddess Pose is a robust and dynamic posture that significantly benefits physical and mental health. It is a favorite in many yoga practices for its empowering and strengthening qualities.

High Lunge Pose also known as Crescent Lunge

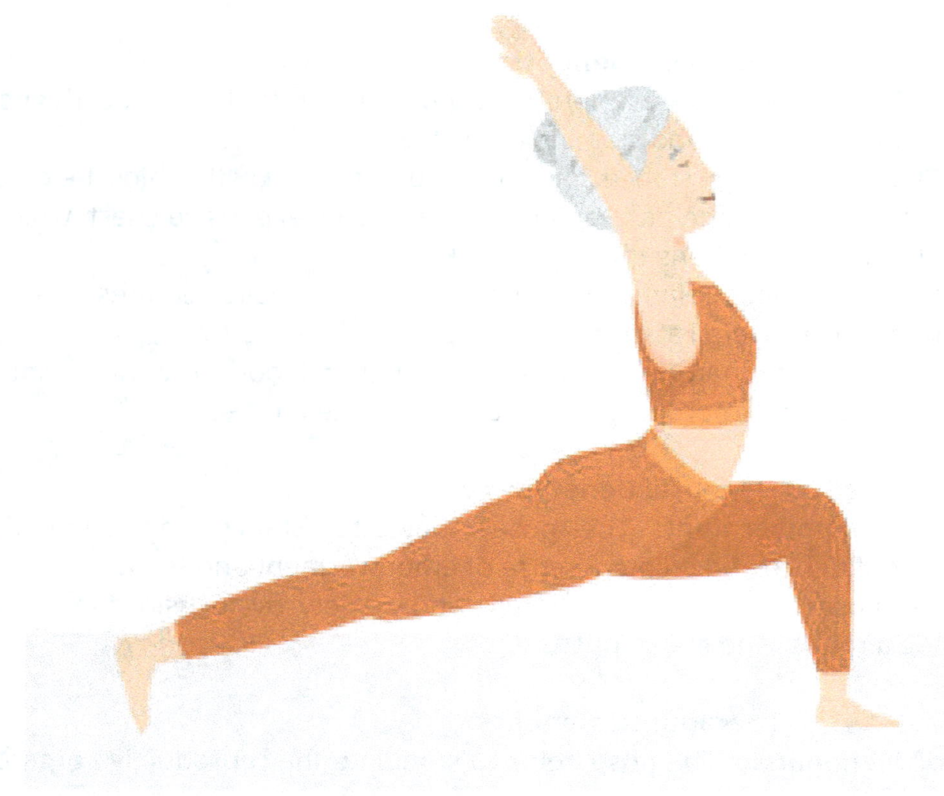

Start Position: Begin in a standing position. Step back about 3 to 4 feet, depending on your comfort and balance.

Align Your Stance: It's crucial to keep your front knee bent directly over the ankle. Your back leg is straight and robust, with the heel lifted off the floor, maintaining a balanced posture.

Torso and Arms: Keep your torso upright. Raise your arms overhead for balance, or place your hands on your hips if that feels more stable.

Engage Core: It's essential to draw your navel towards your spine to stabilize your core, which is the key to maintaining balance in this pose.

Hold and Breathe: Hold the pose for 3 to 5 breaths, focusing on a steady, even breath.

To Release: Step your back foot forward to return to a standing position. Repeat on the opposite side.

Chair Support:
Place a sturdy chair in front of you. Step one foot back and keep the other forward, bending the front knee to a comfortable angle. Rest your hands on the back of the chair for balance. This modification helps maintain stability and reduces the load on the legs.

Block for Balance:
Use a yoga block on either side of the front foot. This allows you to rest your hands on the blocks instead of reaching the floor, reducing strain on your back and maintaining better balance.

Wall Support:
Perform the pose near a wall. You can use the wall to steady yourself with one hand, which is especially helpful for maintaining balance while focusing on the alignment of the legs and hips.

Shallow Lunge:
Reduce the distance between your feet instead of stepping back into a deep lunge. A shallower lunge reduces strain on the knee and hip of the back leg, making the pose more comfortable.

Reduced Back Leg Extension:
Rather than fully extending the back leg, you can keep a slight bend in the knee to avoid over-straining the joints. This also helps maintain balance and stability.

Foot Alignment:
If it feels more natural and comfortable, keep the back foot slightly turned out rather than pointing straight back. This adjustment can help maintain balance and reduce the back leg's hip stress.

Advantages of practicing High Lunge Pose

Physical Benefits:
Strengthens the Lower Body: High Lunge Pose intensely works the muscles of the legs, including the quadriceps, hamstrings, calves, and glutes. It helps build strength and stamina in these areas.
Improves Balance and Stability: Balancing in the high lunge requires and enhances core stability and overall balance, which are crucial for everyday activities and athletic performance.
Increases Hip Flexibility: The pose involves a deep stretch in the hip flexors of the back leg and the hips of the front leg, promoting greater flexibility and range of motion.
Enhances Core Strength: Maintaining the upright position in a High Lunge necessitates engaging the abdominal muscles, thereby strengthening the core.
Stretches the Spine: The upright posture and slight backbend involved in some variations of High Lunge help lengthen and stretch the spine.

Mental Benefits:
Improves Focus and Concentration: Holding a challenging pose like High Lunge requires focus and mental clarity, which can enhance attention-related cognitive functions.
Boosts Energy and Vitality: High Lunge is an invigorating pose that increases circulation and energy flow throughout the body, reducing fatigue and boosting vitality.

Therapeutic Benefits:
Alleviates Sciatica: By stretching and strengthening the muscles around the lower spine and hips, High Lunge can help relieve some of the discomfort associated with sciatica.
Improves Digestive Health: The engagement of core muscles and the overall dynamic nature of the pose stimulate abdominal organs, aiding digestion and metabolism.

Caution:
People with knee or hip issues should approach High Lunge with caution. Modifications can be made, such as adjusting the depth of the lunge or using props like blocks to support the hands if they do not comfortably reach the ground.

High Lunge Pose is a versatile and beneficial posture that supports a wide range of fitness and wellness goals. It is popular in many yoga sequences for its strength-building, balancing, and energizing effects.

Baddha Konasana (Bound Angle Pose)

Start Seated: Sit with a straight spine on a cushion or folded blanket, which will provide a comfortable and supportive base for your hips.

Position Legs: Bend your knees to bring the soles of your feet together in front of you, creating a diamond shape with your legs. If your hips feel tight, keep your feet away from your body.

Support Knees: Place folded blankets or blocks under each knee for support if they don't comfortably reach the floor.

Hand Placement: Hold your feet or ankles. If this feels uncomfortable, you can place your hands on the floor beside your hips for support.

Maintain Posture: Inhale to lengthen your spine. Exhale and gently hinge forward from your hips, leading with your chest, to deepen the stretch without straining. Keep your back straight.

Hold and Breathe: Stay in the pose for 1-3 minutes, focusing on deep, slow breaths. This will help you relax further into the stretch with each exhale, enhancing the pose's benefits.

Release: To come out, release your hands, use your hands to lift your knees, and straighten your legs.

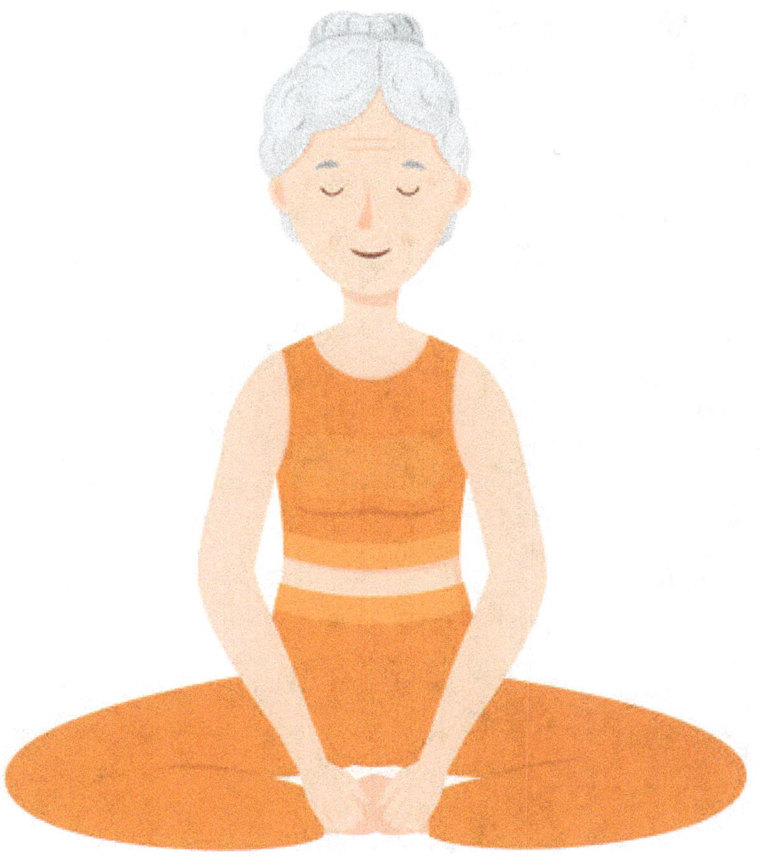

Modifications for Seniors

Cushion Support:
Sit on a cushion or a folded blanket to elevate the hips. This helps tilt the pelvis forward, making it easier to maintain an upright spine and reducing strain on the hips and lower back.

Prop Under Knees:
Place folded towels, yoga blocks, or cushions under each knee or thigh. This support can alleviate pressure on the hips and help those with tight hips or knees to maintain the pose more comfortably.

Wall Support:
Sit with your back against a wall. The wall supports the back, helping keep the spine straight and reducing the effort needed to hold the upper body upright.

Hand Position:
Instead of trying to grasp the feet or toes, which might be challenging, place the hands on the ankles or rest them on the thighs. This lessens the forward lean and helps maintain balance and stability.

Seated Chair Modification:
If sitting on the floor is too difficult, perform Baddha Konasana while seated on a chair. Sit on the edge of the chair and place each foot on additional chairs or sturdy supports so the legs form a diamond shape. This allows you to experience the hip-opening benefits without the strain of sitting on the floor.

Key benefits of practicing Baddha Konasana

Physical Benefits:

Improves Hip and Groin Flexibility: Baddha Konasana is excellent for opening the hips and increasing the range of motion in the groin and hip joints. This is particularly beneficial for those who sit for long periods or have tight hips.

Stretches the Inner Thighs: The pose provides a deep stretch to the muscles of the inner thighs, which can help alleviate tightness and improve leg flexibility.

Stimulates Abdominal Organs: The forward bend in this pose can apply gentle pressure on the abdomen, stimulating the organs within. This stimulation can help improve digestion and the functioning of reproductive organs.

Promotes Pelvic and Lower Back Health: Regular practice of this pose can strengthen the muscles of the lower back and improve the stability of the pelvic region, which is beneficial for posture and overall back health.

Mental Benefits:

Reduces Stress and Anxiety: The seated, meditative nature of Baddha Konasana helps to calm the mind, reducing feelings of stress and anxiety.

Enhances Focus and Calm: As with many yoga poses, focusing on breath and posture during Baddha Konasana can improve mental clarity and focus.

Therapeutic Benefits:

Relieves Menstrual Discomfort and Menopause Symptoms: The opening of the hips and the gentle pressure on the abdomen can help alleviate discomfort associated with menstruation and menopause.

Beneficial for Prostate Health: Stimulating the pelvic region is also helpful for maintaining prostate health and can help alleviate symptoms of urinary disorders.

Additional Benefits:

Facilitates Childbirth: For pregnant women, practicing Baddha Konasana can help prepare the hips and pelvic muscles for childbirth. However, it should be practiced cautiously and possibly under supervision as the pregnancy progresses.

Improves Circulation in the Lower Body: The position of the legs and the gentle forward bend can help improve blood circulation in the lower body.

Caution:

While Baddha Konasana is generally safe, it should be practiced with care by those with knee or hip issues. Using cushions or blocks under the thighs can help reduce strain on these joints if the stretch feels too intense.

Overall, Baddha Konasana is a versatile and beneficial yoga pose that supports physical and mental health, making it a valuable addition to many yoga practices.

Paschimottanasana (Seated Forward Bend)

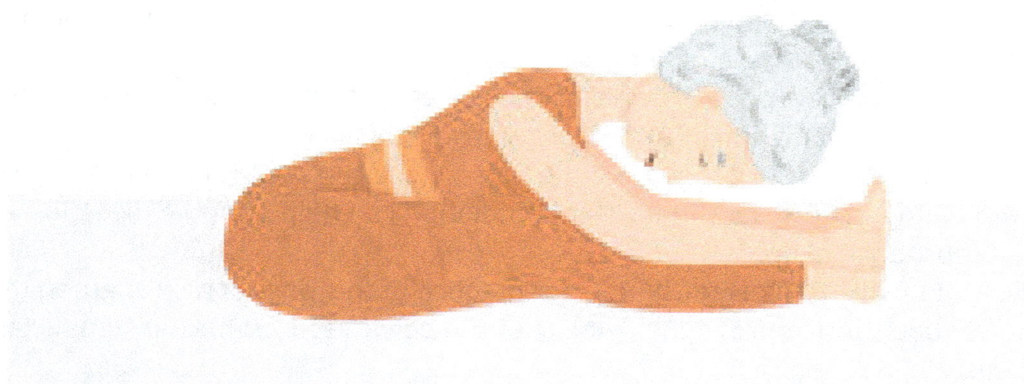

Start Seated: Begin seated on the floor with your legs extended straight in front of you. If flexibility allows, keep your feet together; otherwise, a slight separation is fine.

Sit Up Tall: Inhale and lengthen your spine. Sit up tall, reaching the crown of your head towards the ceiling.

Hinge Forward: Exhale and hinge from your hips to lean forward. Extend your hands towards your feet. Remember, the goal is not to touch your toes but to feel a comfortable stretch along your back and the back of your legs.

Maintain Alignment: Keep your spine as straight as possible, leading with your chest rather than rounding your back. This ensures a deeper and safer stretch.

Hold and Breathe: Hold the position for a few breaths, deepening the stretch with each exhale. Avoid straining; focus on a gentle stretch.

To Release: Inhale and gently come back up to a seated position.

Benefits of practicing Paschimottanasana:

Physical Benefits:
Stretches the Hamstrings and Lower Back: One of Paschimottanasana's primary benefits is its deep stretch of the hamstrings and lower back muscles, which can help alleviate tightness and improve flexibility in these areas.
Calms the Spinal Nerves: The forward bend helps elongate and relieve tension along the spine, soothing the spinal nerves and promoting a healthy spine.
Stimulates Abdominal Organs: The folding action compresses the abdominal organs, enhancing blood flow to these areas and stimulating the kidneys, liver, ovaries, and uterus, which can help improve the functionality of these organs.
Improves Digestion: Compressing the abdomen against the thighs in this pose can help stimulate digestive function and alleviate problems such as constipation.

Mental Benefits:
Relieves Stress: The forward bend's introspective nature can calm the mind, helping to reduce stress and anxiety.
Enhances Focus and Concentration: Maintaining the pose requires a degree of mental focus, which can help improve overall concentration and clarity of thought.

Therapeutic Benefits:
Alleviates Menstrual Discomfort and Menopause Symptoms: For women, the pose can help relieve the symptoms associated with menstruation and menopause by soothing the abdominal and pelvic regions.
Beneficial for Hypertension: The calming effect of the pose on the nervous system can help lower blood pressure and reduce symptoms of hypertension. However, those with severe cases should proceed with caution and under guidance.

Caution:
Back Issues: Individuals with back injuries should practice this pose cautiously, possibly avoiding deep forward bends or practicing a modified version with a slight knee bend.
Hernia: Those with a hernia should avoid deep forward bends that pressure the abdomen.
Pregnancy: Pregnant women should modify the pose to avoid compressing the abdomen, typically by keeping the legs slightly apart or performing the pose under the guidance of a qualified instructor.
Paschimottanasana is a comprehensive pose that profoundly benefits overall health and well-being, making it a staple in many yoga practices. However, due to its intensity, it's essential to approach the pose gradually and properly to maximize its benefits and minimize the risk of injury.

Day 3

Manipura Chakra
Its element is Fire

The Manipura Chakra Located around the navel area and extending up to the breastbone, it is the center of personal power, self-esteem, and confidence.

Signs of a Balanced:
A strong sense of personal power and autonomy
High self-esteem and confidence
The ability to make decisions and meet challenges
Healthy digestion and metabolism

Signs of Imbalance:
Excessive control and power over others, aggression
Low self-esteem, feeling powerless or victimized
Indecisiveness, fear of confrontation
Digestive issues, such as ulcers, heartburn, eating disorders, or indigestion

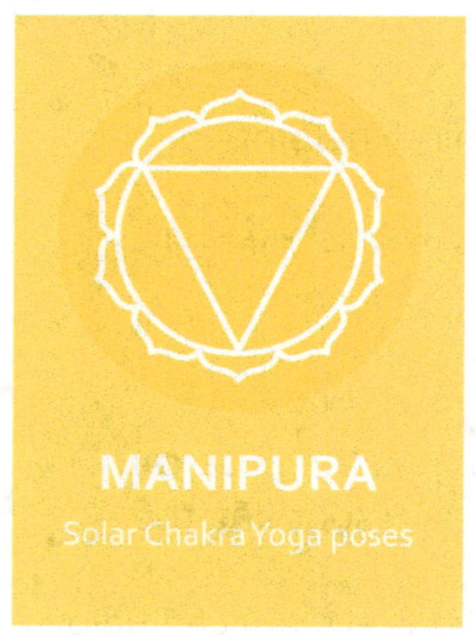

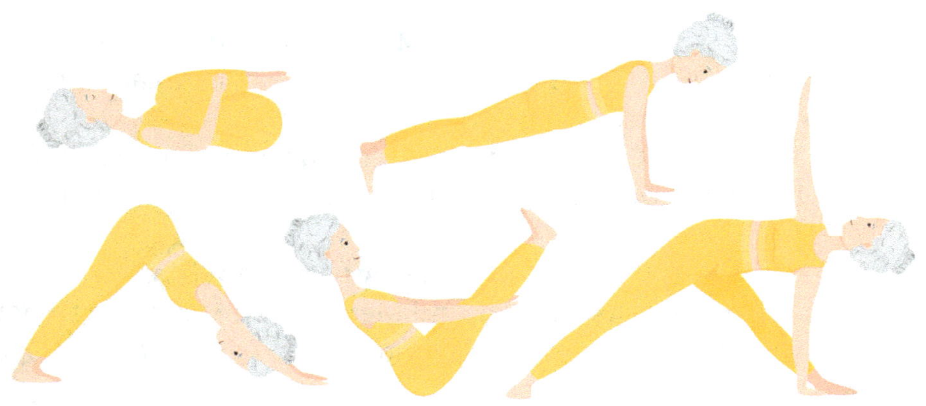

Mindfulness and Affirmations:
Positive affirmations that reinforce personal power and self-worth, such as
"I am strong and brave" or
"I trust my intuition and wisdom,"

Pranayama:
Breathing exercises that generate heat, such as Kapalabhati (Skull Shining Breath) and Bhastrika (Bellows Breath), can stimulate and balance this energy center.

Meditation:
Visualizing a bright yellow light or flame in the solar plexus area can help clear blockages and stimulate this chakra. Focusing on the seed mantra "Ram" during meditation can also be effective.

Adho Mukha Svanasana – Downward–Facing Dog Pose

To revisit the instructions for this pose, please refer to page 33.

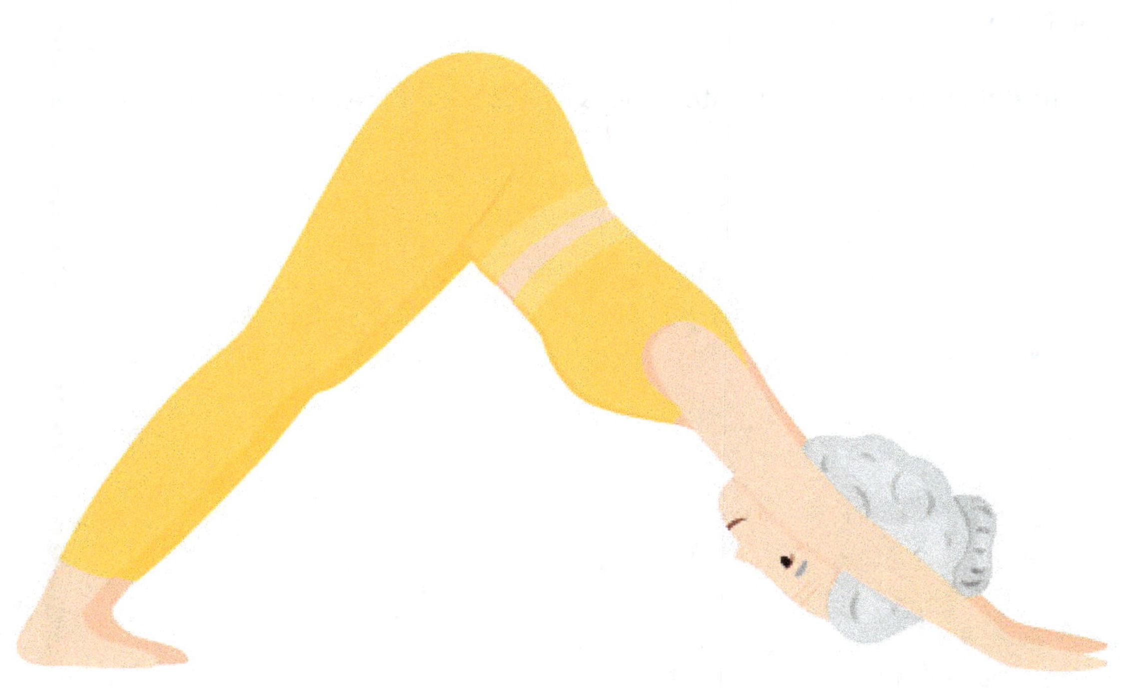

Phalakasana, also the Plank Pose.

Leg Movement: Inhale and extend your left leg back, straightening your torso into a plank position.

Arm Alignment: Ensure your arms are perpendicular to the floor, providing vital support.

Gaze and Spine: Keep your gaze forward and ensure your spine remains straight, forming a straight line from your head to your heels.

Stability and Relaxation: Maintain steadiness in this position while remaining relaxed.

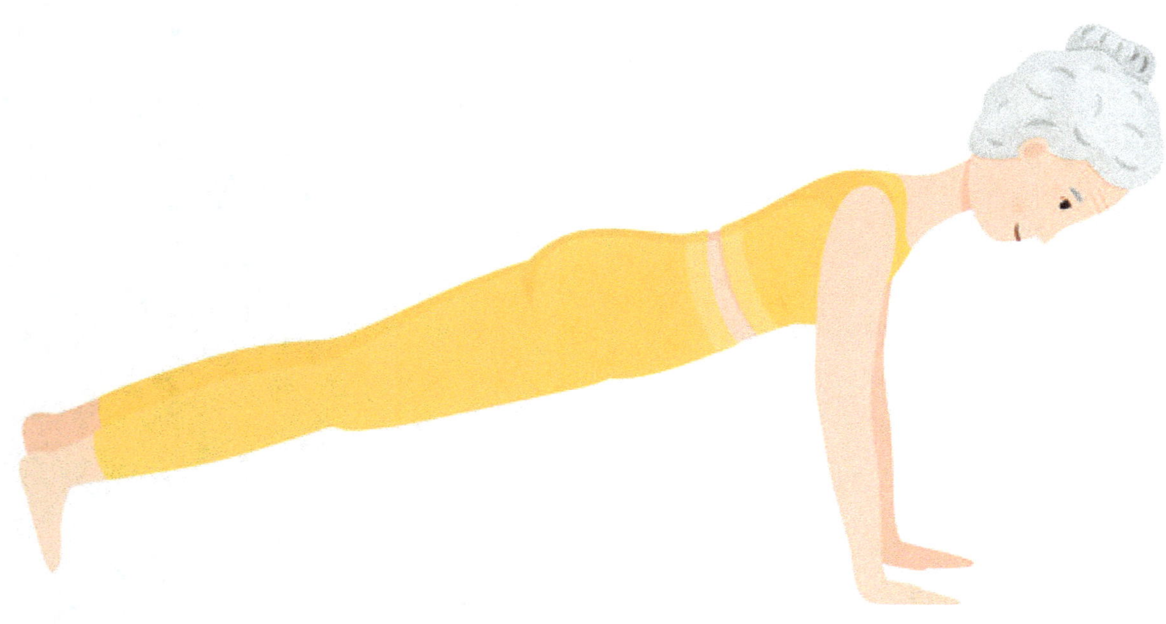

Knees Down Plank:
Begin in a standard plank position, but lower your knees to the ground. Keep your core engaged and ensure your back remains straight from your head to your knees. This modification reduces the core and upper body strain while strengthening these areas.

Forearm Plank:
Instead of extending your arms straight with hands flat on the ground, lower onto your forearms. This position can be less strenuous on the wrists and shoulders. You can also do this version with knees down for additional support.

Wall Plank:
Stand facing a wall, approximately an arm's length away. Place your hands on the wall at shoulder height. Walk your feet back until your body forms a straight line from head to heels, leaning into the wall. This version significantly reduces the load on the core and lower body, making it much easier to maintain.

Chair Plank:
Place your hands on the seat of a sturdy chair, stepping your feet back so your body forms a straight line from your head to your heels, similar to the wall plank. This modification is more accessible than a floor plank but effectively engages the core and upper body muscles.

Incline Plank:
Use a raised surface like a sturdy bench or the edge of a bed for your hands. The higher the surface, the less intense the plank. This version helps gradually build core strength without the full intensity of a floor plank.

Benefits of practicing Plank Pose

Physical Benefits:
Strengthens the Core: One of the primary benefits of Phalakasana is its ability to build core strength. The pose engages the deep core muscles, including the transversus abdominis, obliques, and rectus abdominis, enhancing stability and core endurance.
Enhances Upper Body Strength: Plank Pose requires you to support your body weight with your arms, shoulders, and chest, strengthening these areas along with the upper back.
Builds Lower Body Stamina: The pose also engages the leg muscles, including the quadriceps and calves, as you work to maintain a stable, straight line from head to heels.
Improves Posture: Regular practice of Phalakasana can help improve overall posture by strengthening the spine, shoulders, and pelvic muscles, essential for maintaining proper alignment and balance.
Increases Metabolic Rate: As a full-body exercise, Plank Pose can help boost metabolism by increasing muscle mass, which burns more calories even at rest.

Mental Benefits:
Enhances Focus and Concentration: Maintaining the pose requires mental focus to hold the body steady and aligned, which can improve overall mental concentration and discipline.
Reduces Stress: Like many physical exercises, Plank Pose can help reduce stress by increasing endorphin production, the body's natural painkillers and mood elevators.

Therapeutic Benefits:
Alleviates Back Pain: By strengthening the core, Plank Pose can help relieve pressure on the spine, supporting better spine health and reducing symptoms of lower back pain.
Promotes Bone and Joint Health: Engaging in weight-bearing exercises like Plank Pose can help strengthen bones and joints, crucial for preventing osteoporosis and reducing the risk of joint degeneration.

Caution:
While Plank Pose is generally safe for most people, those with wrist, elbow, or shoulder problems should proceed cautiously. To reduce strain on the wrists, the pose can be modified by performing it on the forearms.
Phalakasana is a versatile and beneficial pose that supports physical fitness, mental clarity, and overall health, making it a valuable addition to any exercise routine.

Triangle Pose, or Trikonasana,

Start by standing wide on your mat, with feet about 3-4 feet apart. Extend arms parallel to the floor.

Position Feet: Turn your right foot out 90 degrees and your left foot in slightly. Align the heels.

Enter Pose: Exhale and hinge at the right hip to extend the torso over the right leg. Place the right hand on the shin, ankle, or the floor. Stretch the left arm vertically, aligning it with the shoulders.

Gaze: Look up towards your left hand, or keep the neck neutral if more comfortable.

Hold: Maintain for 30 seconds to 1 minute, breathing steadily.

Release: Inhale to rise, reverse foot direction, and repeat on the opposite side.

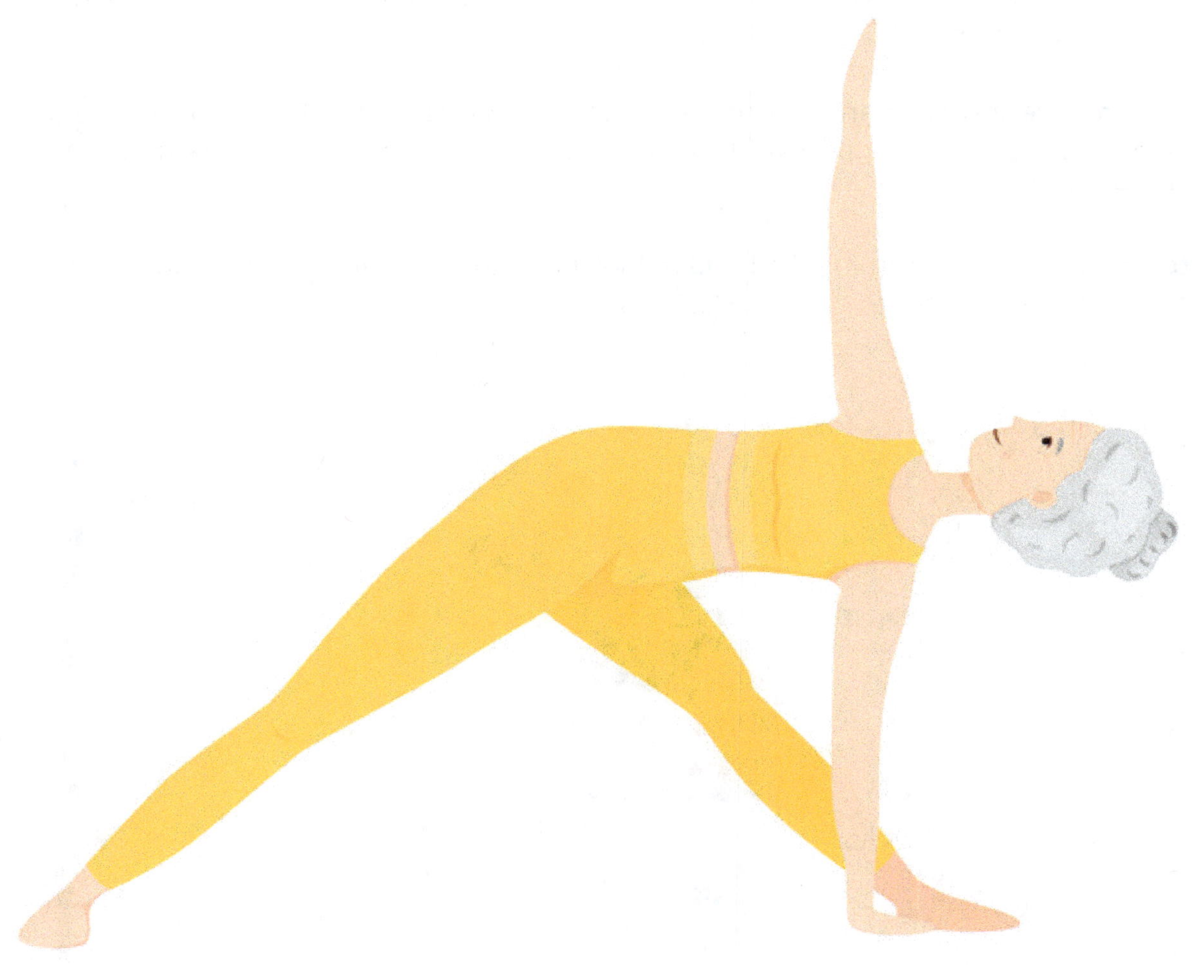

Modifications to make Triangle Pose more accessible:

Use of Props:
Yoga Block: Place a yoga block on the inside or outside of the front foot. This allows you to rest your hand on the block instead of reaching the floor, reducing strain on the balance and flexibility of the torso.

Chair: Use a chair placed outside the front leg. Rest your hand on the seat of the chair. This modification significantly reduces the need for bending sideways and helps maintain balance.

Shorten the Stance: Reduce the distance between your feet. This straightforward modification makes it easier to balance and reduces the stretch required in the hamstrings and hips, giving you a sense of reassurance and confidence in your practice.

Hand Position: Instead of extending the lower hand towards the floor or block, place it on your shin or thigh. This adjustment decreases the intensity of the bend and still allows for a good stretch along the side of the body.
The upper hand can also be placed on the hip instead of extending it towards the ceiling to reduce shoulder strain.

Wall Support: Perform a Triangle Pose with your back against a wall. This helps ensure proper alignment and provides a supportive structure that makes maintaining balance throughout the pose more accessible.

Gentle Twist: Instead of turning the head to look up at the top hand, seniors can look straight ahead or down at the floor to avoid neck strain.

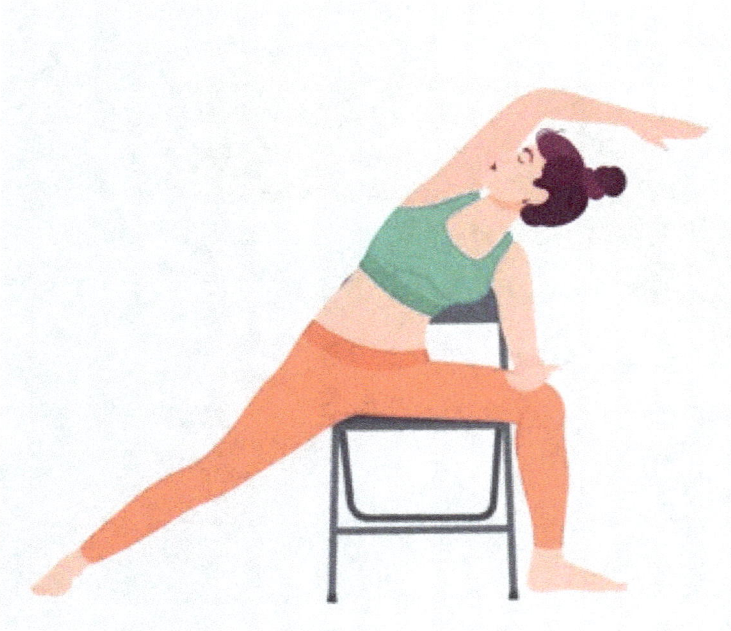

Key benefits of practicing Triangle Pose:

Strengthens Muscles: Triangle Pose engages and strengthens the legs, particularly the thighs and calves. It also works the muscles of the hips, back, and arms, helping to build overall body strength.

Unleashing Flexibility: This pose liberates several body parts, including the hips, groin, hamstrings, and shoulders. Regular practice can lead to greater freedom in your movements and an expanded range of motion.

Stimulates Organs: The twisting nature of Triangle Pose helps stimulate abdominal organs, which can improve digestion and aid in detoxification.

Relieving Stress: The concentration required to maintain balance and alignment in this pose helps focus the mind, offering a soothing relief from stress and anxiety.

Enhances Balance and Stability: Triangle Pose challenges and promotes balance and stability, which are crucial for aging bodies and overall mobility.

Therapeutic for Back Pain: Triangle Pose can strengthen and stretch the spine, Which can be therapeutic for people with back pain, mainly when performed with proper alignment and modifications if necessary.

Increases Mental Focus: Holding the pose and maintaining the correct alignment requires concentration and mental focus, which can enhance cognitive functions.

Opens the Chest and Shoulders: It helps open the chest and shoulders, which is beneficial for those who spend long hours sitting, leading to improved breathing and relief from tension in these areas.

Boat Pose or Navasana

Start Position: Begin by sitting on the floor with your knees bent and feet flat. Keep your spine straight and hands resting beside your hips.

Enter the Pose: Lean back slightly, find balance on your sit bones, and lift your feet off the floor. Initially, you can keep the knees bent. If you feel stable, straighten your legs to form a V-shape with your body. Extend your arms forward, parallel to the floor, palms facing each other.

Alignment: Keep your chest open and your spine as straight as possible. Engage your core muscles to maintain balance. Look straight ahead to keep the neck in a neutral position.

Hold and Breathe: Hold the pose for 3-5 breaths, gradually increasing the duration as you gain strength and stability. This gradual increase is important to avoid strain and encourage steady progress. Keep breathing smoothly throughout the pose.

Release: To come out of the pose, lower your feet to the floor on an exhale and relax in a seated position.

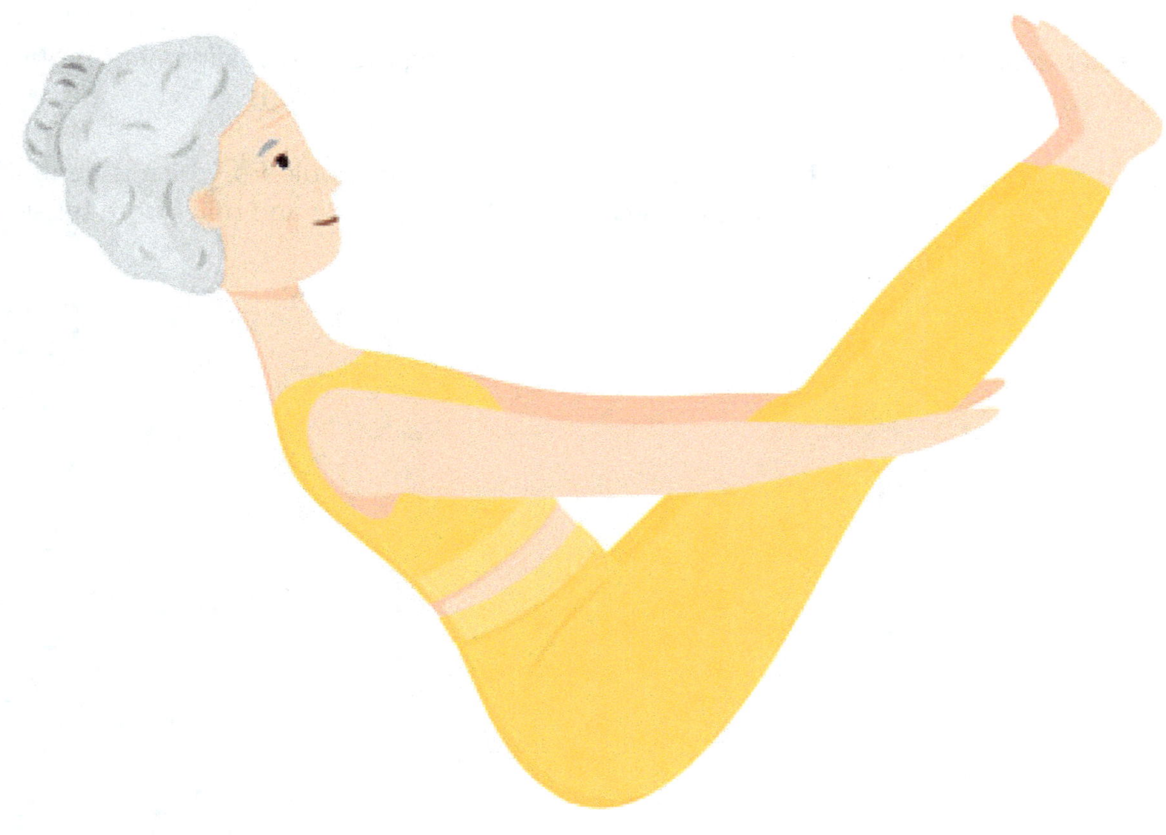

Modifications for Seniors

Keeping Knees Bent: If straightening the legs is too challenging, you can perform Navasana with your knees bent. This variation still strengthens the core without putting too much strain on the lower back.

Support With Hands: If balancing is difficult, you can place your hands on the floor behind your hips for support. Gradually try to lift one hand at a time off the floor to increase the challenge as you become more comfortable.

Chair Variation: To adapt Navasana for chair yoga, sit on the edge of a chair without arms. Lean back slightly, holding onto the sides of the chair for balance. Lift your legs, keeping knees bent, to a comfortable height. This variation engages the core while providing stability and support.

Benefits of practicing Navasana:

Physical Benefits:

Strengthens the Core: Boat Pose intensely works the deep core muscles, including the abdominals and the muscles around the spine, which are essential for overall stability and balance.

Improves Digestion: Holding the pose can stimulate the abdominal organs, including the kidneys, intestines, and thyroid, which can help improve digestion and metabolism.

Enhances Hip Flexor Strength: Navasana requires you to keep your legs lifted, which engages and strengthens the hip flexors and muscles of the lower abdomen.

Strengthens the Spine: Maintaining the V-shape posture helps strengthen the muscles along the spine, improving posture and potentially alleviating back pain.

Mental Benefits:

Increases Focus and Concentration: Holding the pose requires concentration and mental stamina, which can help enhance overall mental clarity and focus.

Builds Willpower and Discipline: The challenging nature of Boat Pose requires and develops willpower, discipline, and determination as you strive to maintain the pose for more extended periods.

Therapeutic Benefits:

Stimulates the Thyroid and Kidneys: By improving circulation to the abdominal region, Navasana can help enhance the functioning of the thyroid and kidneys, contributing to better overall health.

Alleviates Stress: Although physically demanding, the intense focus can help divert attention from daily stressors, providing a mental break and reducing overall stress levels.

Caution:

While Navasana is beneficial, it should be approached with caution, especially by those with low back pain or issues, as it can exacerbate such conditions. Pregnant women should avoid this pose or modify it under the guidance of a qualified instructor. People with heart problems or high blood pressure should also practice with caution.

Navasana is a powerful pose that builds physical and mental strength, promotes health, and enhances overall vitality, making it a valued addition to many yoga practices.

Apanasana, often called the "Knees-to-Chest Pose"

Start Position: Begin by lying on your back on a comfortable, flat surface. Keep your legs extended and arms at your sides, palms facing down.

Enter the Pose: On an exhale, gently draw both knees toward your chest. Wrap your arms around your shins just below the knees. If it's comfortable for you, interlace your fingers or hold onto each elbow with the opposite hand.

Alignment: Keep your back flat on the floor. You can place a small, folded towel under your sacrum for support if there's a significant arch in your lower back.

Hold and Breathe: Hold this position for 1-3 minutes, breathing deeply and evenly. With each exhale, allow your body to relax more deeply, releasing tension in your back and abdomen.

Release: To come out of the pose, release your legs and gently lower your feet to the floor. Extend your legs and rest for a few moments before moving on to your next activity.

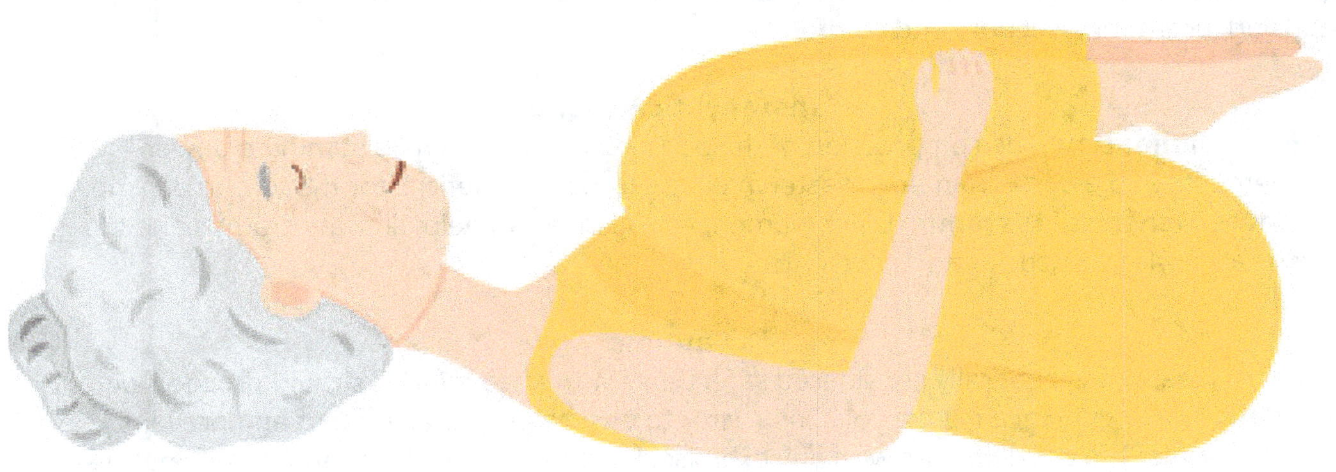

One Leg at a Time: If bringing both knees to the chest is too challenging, you can modify the pose by drawing one knee at a time toward the chest while keeping the other leg extended on the floor or bent with the foot on the floor.

Use of Props: Placing a cushion or folded blanket under your head can provide additional neck support. If you find it difficult to reach your legs, you can also use a yoga strap around your shins.

Physical Benefits:

Relieves Lower Back Pain: Apanasana helps alleviate tension and discomfort in this area by gently stretching the lower back. It's particularly beneficial for those who sit for long periods or suffer from chronic lower back issues.

Improves Digestion: The compression of the abdomen against the thighs in this pose stimulates abdominal organs, including the intestines and liver, which can help enhance digestion and relieve gas and bloating.

Stretches the Hips and Thighs: Although a gentle pose, Apanasana provides a light stretch to the hip joints and muscles of the thigh, which can improve flexibility and reduce stiffness.

Promotes Relaxation: The pose has a natural calming effect on the body, promoting relaxation and reducing symptoms of stress.

Mental Benefits:

Calms the Mind: The soothing nature of the pose, combined with focused breathing, helps calm the mind and reduce anxiety and mental stress.

Enhances Emotional Release: Drawing the knees to the chest can help release emotional tension, promoting security and comfort.

Therapeutic Benefits:

Aids in Elimination: The compression of the abdominal area can help stimulate bowel movements and aid in eliminating waste, making this pose beneficial for those with constipation.

Relieves Menstrual Discomfort: For women, Apanasana can help alleviate cramps and bloating associated with menstruation.

Caution:

While Apanasana is generally considered safe, those with knee injuries should proceed with caution or seek guidance from a yoga instructor to ensure proper alignment and prevent aggravation of the condition. As with any exercise, listening to your body and modifying the pose to accommodate any physical limitations is essential.

Overall, Apanasana is a beneficial yoga pose that offers relaxation and physical relief. It is a valuable addition to a yoga practice, especially as a gentle way to wind down or as a preparatory pose for more profound relaxation or sleep.

Day 4
Anahata, or the Heart Chakra
Its element is Air

Located in the center of the chest at the heart level, it acts as the individual's center of compassion, empathy, love, and forgiveness.

Signs of a Balanced :
Feeling open and accepting of oneself and others
Experiencing deep and meaningful relationships
Possessing a strong sense of empathy and compassion
Demonstrating patience and understanding

Signs of an Imbalance:
Difficulty in relationships, feeling isolated
Holding onto grudges, inability to forgive
Experiencing feelings of unworthiness
Over-loving to the point of suffocation, or an inability to express love

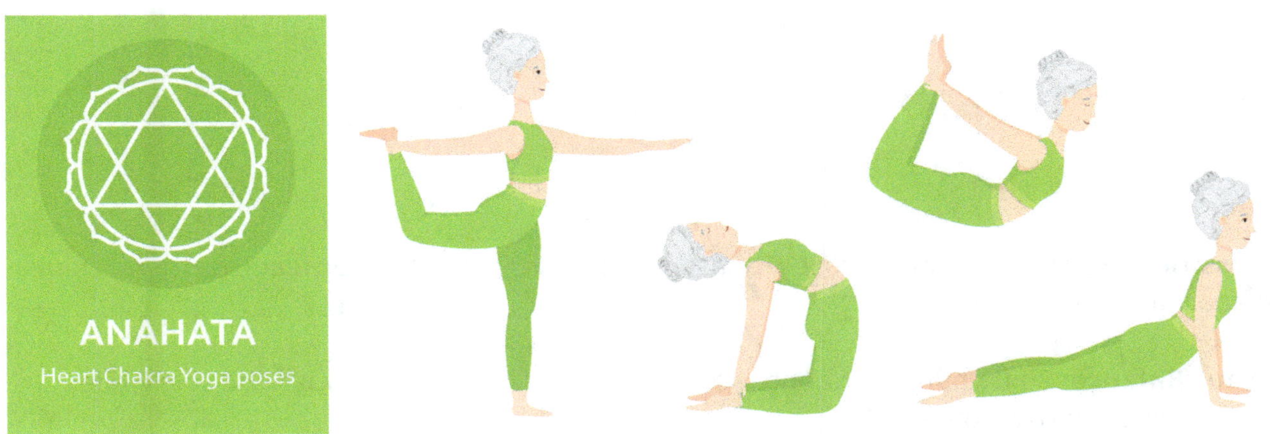

Pranayama:
Breathing exercises like Anulom Vilom (Alternate Nostril Breathing) with a focus on the heart area during inhalation and exhalation can help in clearing blockages and enhancing the flow of energy through Anahata.

Meditation:
Visualizing a bright green or pink light in the heart area while meditating can help in opening and balancing Anahata. Chanting or focusing on the seed mantra "Yam" during meditation is also beneficial.

Mindfulness and Affirmations:"
I am open to love," "I forgive myself and others," and "I live in balance, in a state of gracefulness and gratitude."

Dancer's Pose (Natarajasana)

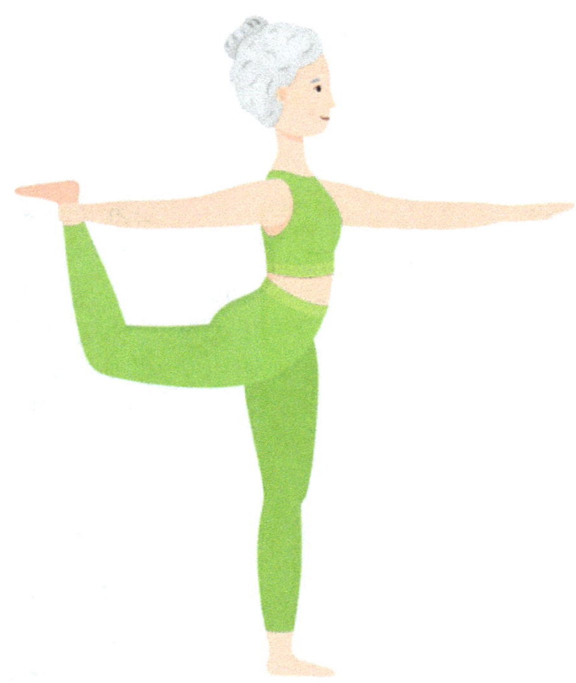

Start Position: Begin in Mountain Pose (Tadasana), standing tall with your feet together or hip-width apart for more stability.

Find Your Balance: Shift your weight onto your right foot, grounding through the sole while slightly bending the right knee.

Grab Your Left Foot: Bend your left knee and reach your left hand backward to grab the outside of your left foot or ankle. If reaching your foot is challenging, loop a yoga strap around your foot and hold the strap with your hand.

Enter the Pose: Extend your right arm forward, palm facing up, as a counterbalance. Inhale, and as you exhale, gently kick your left foot into your hand, lifting the foot up and back, away from your torso. Tilt your torso forward, maintaining balance and strength in the standing leg.

Hold and Breathe: Focus on a spot in front of you to maintain balance. Hold the pose for 3-5 breaths, gradually increasing the lift of your left leg while keeping your hips squared to the front.

To Release: Gently lower your left foot back to the ground, release the grip, and return to Mountain Pose. Repeat on the other side.

Modifications for Seniors or Beginners:

Use a Wall: Stand near a wall, using it for balance as you enter, and hold the pose. You can lightly touch the wall with your free hand.

Chair for Support: Perform the pose standing behind a chair, holding onto the back with your free hand for support.

Yoga Strap: If grabbing your foot is difficult, use a yoga strap looped around the foot being lifted. This allows you to maintain alignment without overstraining.

Keep It Low: Lifting your foot very high is unnecessary. A lower position where you can maintain balance and alignment is more beneficial than straining to lift the leg higher.

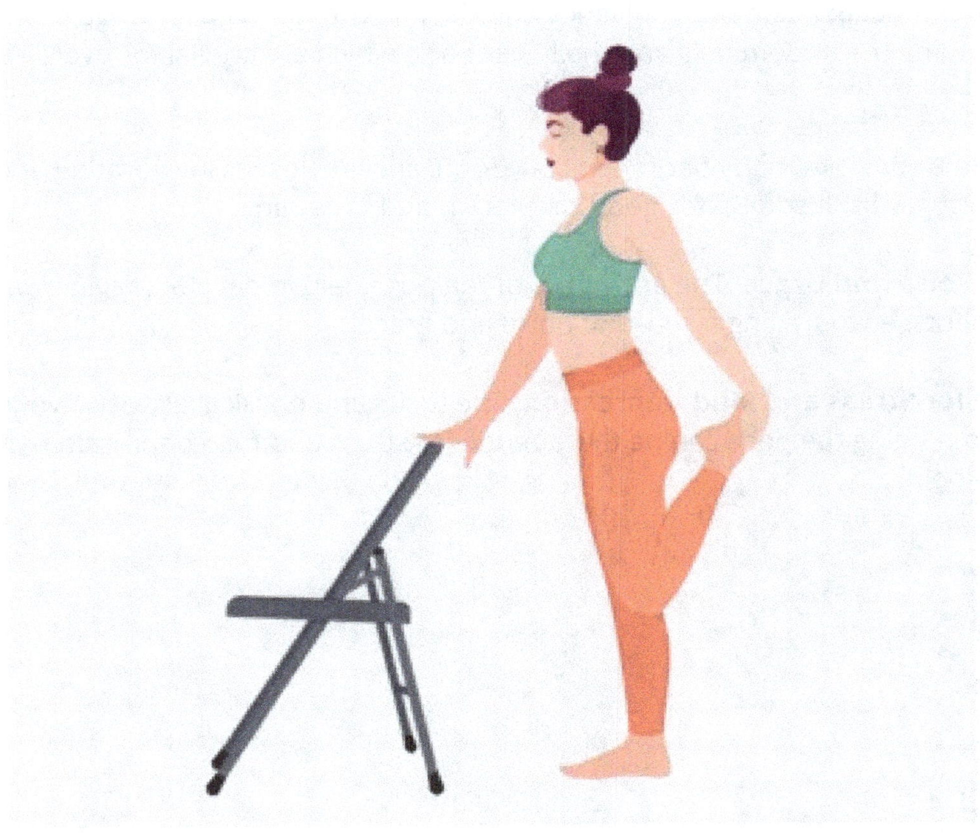

Benefits of practicing Dancer's Pose:

Improves Balance: This pose requires you to stand on one leg, which helps improve your overall balance and stability. Regular practice can enhance your ability to maintain balance in daily activities.

Strengthens the Legs: Supporting the body's weight on one leg significantly strengthens that leg, including the thigh muscles and the supporting muscles around the knee and ankle.

Stretches the Shoulders and Chest: As you reach back to hold your foot, the pose opens up the shoulder joints and stretches the chest, which is beneficial for those who sit for long periods or have poor posture.

Increases Flexibility: Dancer's Pose stretches the hip flexors and the quadriceps of the lifted leg, which can improve flexibility and range of motion in the hips and legs.

Enhances Concentration and Focus: Balancing poses like Dancer's Pose require and cultivate a high level of mental focus and concentration, which can translate into better focus in other areas of life.

Strengthens the Core: Maintaining balance and the integrity of the pose engages the core muscles, including the abdominals and the lower back, which are crucial for overall stability and strength.

Energizes the Body: Like many backbends in yoga, Dancer's Pose is invigorating and can help to increase energy levels. It stimulates good circulation and breathing.

Encourages Poise and Grace: The aesthetics of the pose help in developing an awareness of body movements, encouraging a sense of poise and grace.

Therapeutic for Stress and Mild Depression: The focus and physical activity involved in achieving and holding the pose can be therapeutic for stress and mild depression, promoting a sense of well-being.

Camel Pose (Ustrasana)

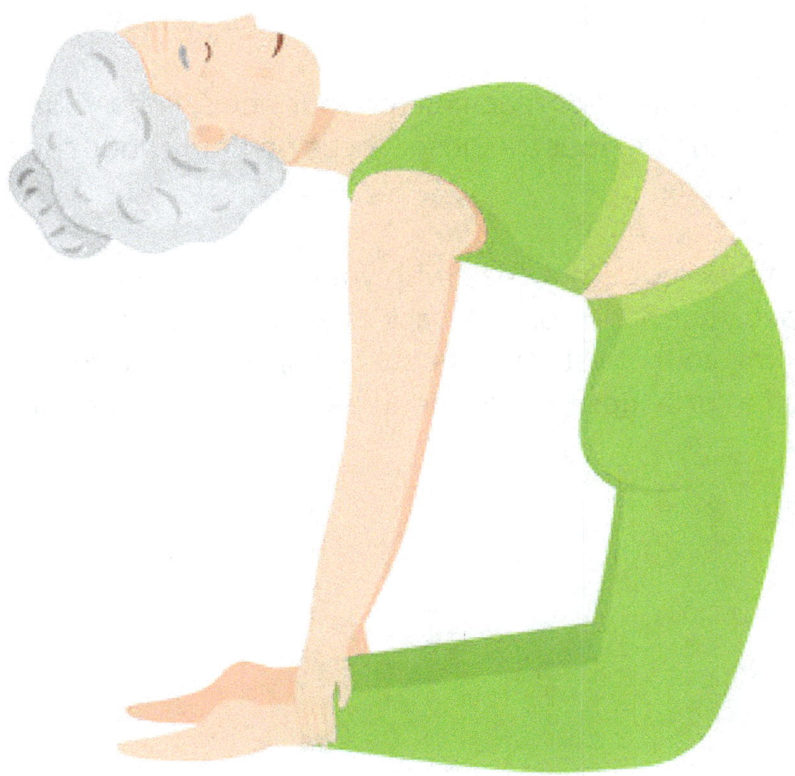

Start Position: Kneel on the yoga mat with your knees hip-width apart and your thighs perpendicular to the floor. Place your hands on your lower back, fingers pointing downwards, elbows, and shoulders drawn back.

Backbend: Inhale deeply, then as you exhale, gently push your hips forward, keeping your thighs vertical. Begin to arch your back, sliding your hands down towards your heels. If possible, reach and hold your heels with your hands.

Head Position: Allow your head to drop back comfortably, opening your throat. If this strains your neck, keep your chin tucked towards your chest instead.

Hold and Breathe: It's important to respect your body's limits. Maintain the pose for a few comfortable breaths, focusing on a gentle stretch in the front of your body and keeping your hips pushed forward. If you feel any discomfort or strain, ease off the pose.

To Release, Inhale, and slowly rise, leading with your chest and keeping your hands on your heels until the last moment. Then, return to the kneeling position.

Modifications for Seniors :

Support with Props: If reaching your heels is challenging, place blocks beside each ankle to reduce the distance. You can also tuck your toes to elevate your heels.

Hands-on Lower Back: Instead of reaching for your heels, keep your hands on your lower back for support throughout the pose. Focus on lifting your chest and a mild backbend without straining.

Chair Support: Sit on the edge of a chair with your feet planted firmly on the ground, hip-width apart. Place your hands on the back of your pelvis. Gently lean back, arching your back and opening your chest towards the ceiling, similar to the action of the Camel Pose. This modification provides the backbend experience with added stability and less intensity.

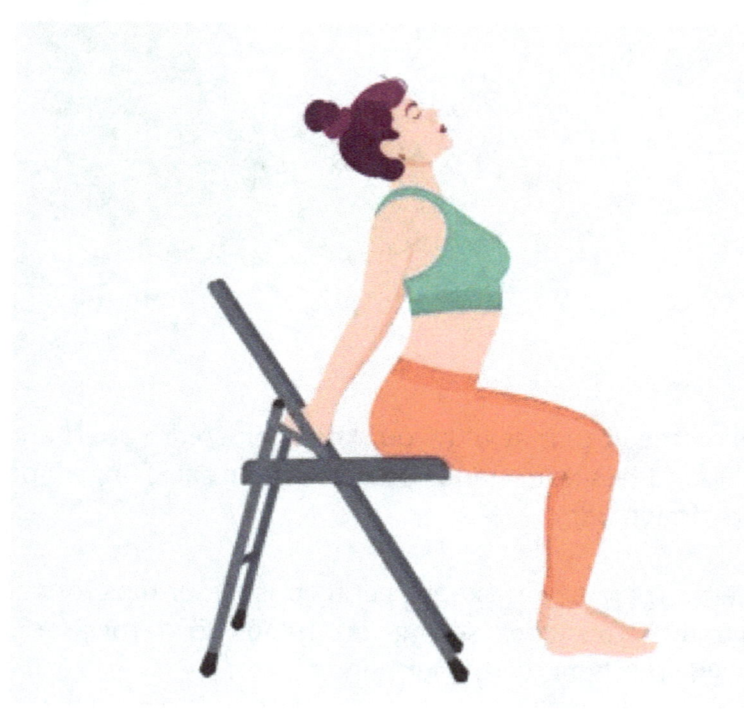

Primary benefits of practicing Camel Pose:

Opens the Front Body: Camel Pose deeply stretches the front of the body, including the chest, abdomen, quadriceps, and hip flexors. This can help counteract the effects of prolonged sitting and forward bending.

Strengthens the Back: This pose engages and strengthens the muscles of the back and shoulders, which are crucial for good posture and spinal health.

Improves Spinal Flexibility: Practicing Ustrasana increases flexibility in the spine, promoting better movement and reducing stiffness. This can be particularly beneficial as part of a regimen to alleviate back pain.

Stimulates Abdominal Organs: The stretch in the abdomen can help stimulate abdominal organs, potentially improving digestion and relieving constipation.

Enhances Thoracic Mobility: Camel Pose helps in opening the thoracic spine (the middle and upper back), which is often stiff. This can improve breathing and relieve respiratory ailments.

Boosts Mood and Energy: As a backbend, Camel Pose is known for its ability to energize the body and uplift the mood. It stimulates the nervous system and can help alleviate mild depression and fatigue.

Improves Posture: By strengthening the back muscles and stretching the front of the body, Camel Pose helps in improving overall posture.

Therapeutic for Anxiety and Stress: The pose's opening effect on the chest and breathing can help relieve anxiety and stress, promoting a sense of well-being.

Promotes Confidence: Backbends like Camel Pose can also help open up the heart center, which is associated with vulnerability and openness, fostering a sense of courage and confidence.

Bhujangasana - Cobra Pose

To revisit the instructions for this pose,
please refer to page 41

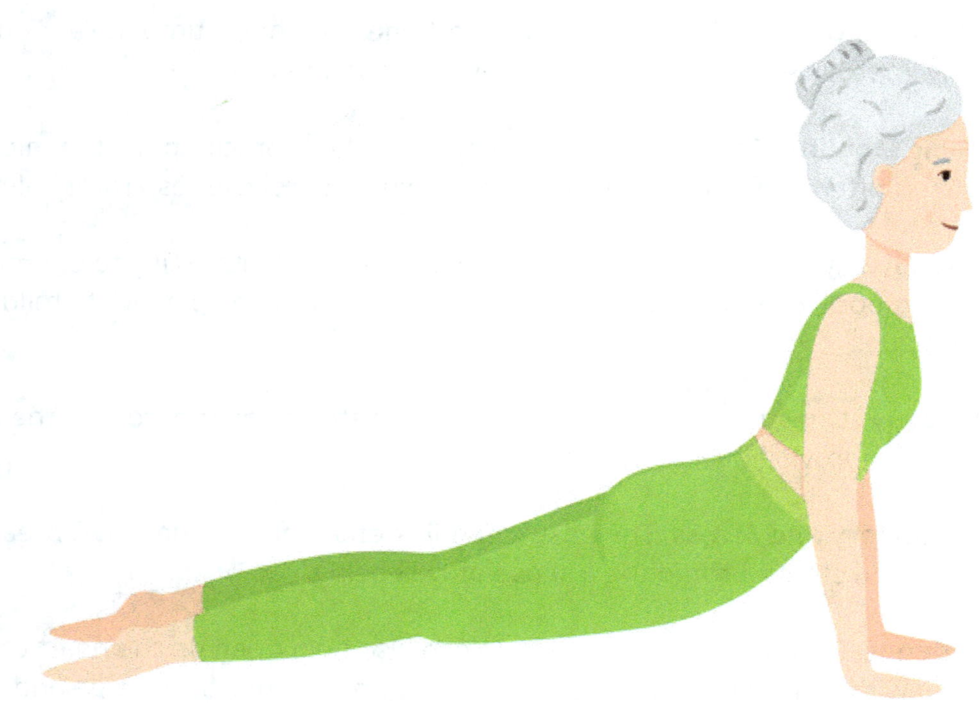

Bow Pose (Dhanurasana)

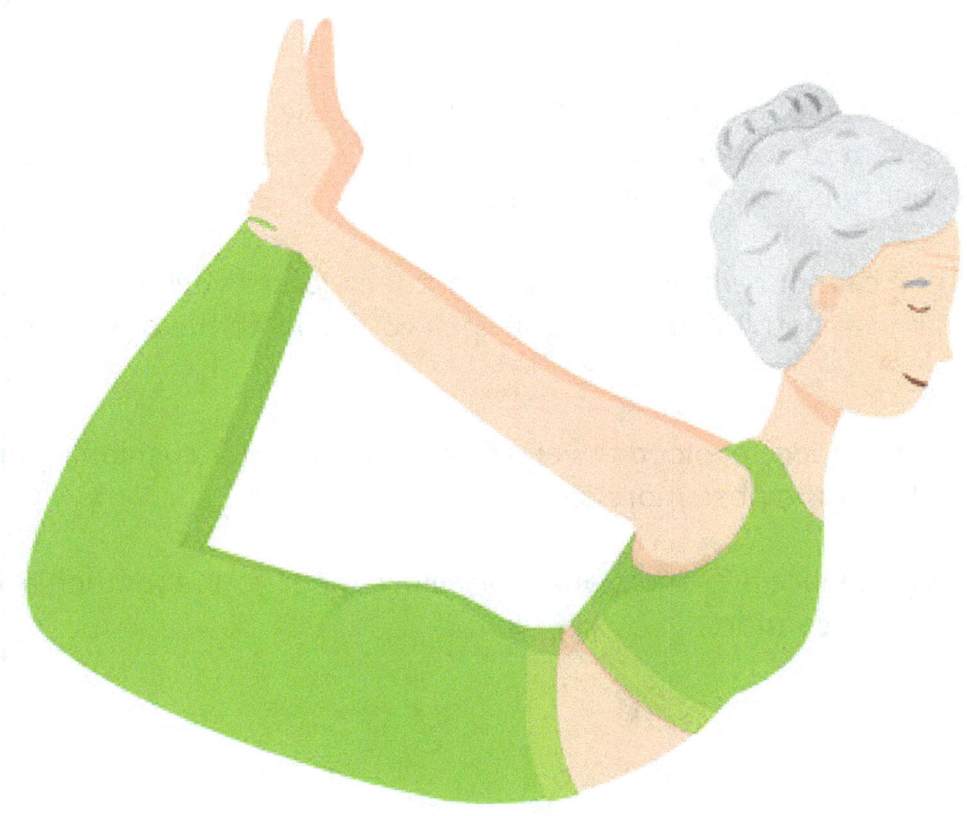

Start Position: Lie flat on your stomach on a yoga mat, with your legs hip-width apart and your arms by your sides.

Grab Your Feet: Bend your knees and reach back to grab the outer edges of your ankles or feet. If catching your feet is difficult, use a yoga strap: loop it around your ankles and hold onto it with both hands, keeping a slight bend in the knees.

Lift: Inhale and lift your chest and knees off the mat by pulling on your ankles or the strap, bringing your body into a bow. Direct your gaze forward to avoid straining the neck.

Hold and Breathe: Maintain the pose for 3-5 breaths, focusing on stretching the front of your body and lifting higher with each inhalation.

To Release: Exhale and gently lower your chest and legs back to the mat. Release your feet or strap, and rest with your head turned to one side.

Half Bow Pose: Instead of lifting both sides simultaneously, work one side at a time. Keep one arm in front of you for balance while bending the opposite leg and reaching back with the other hand to grab your ankle or foot.

Use a Strap: If you cannot comfortably reach your feet, loop a yoga strap around your ankles and hold it with both hands. Gradually pull yourself into the pose without straining.

Towel Under Thighs: Place a folded towel under your thighs for cushioning and support, making lifting the pose more accessible.

Pillow Under Pelvis: Place a folded blanket or pillow under your abdomen to reduce pressure and increase comfort.

Primary benefits of practicing Camel Pose:

Opens the Front Body: Camel Pose deeply stretches the front of the body, including the chest, abdomen, quadriceps, and hip flexors. This can help counteract the effects of prolonged sitting and forward bending.

Strengthens the Back: This pose engages and strengthens the muscles of the back and shoulders, which are crucial for good posture and spinal health.

Improves Spinal Flexibility: Practicing Ustrasana increases flexibility in the spine, promoting better movement and reducing stiffness. This can be particularly beneficial as part of a regimen to alleviate back pain.

Stimulates Abdominal Organs: The stretch in the abdomen can help stimulate abdominal organs, potentially improving digestion and relieving constipation.

Enhances Thoracic Mobility: Camel Pose helps in opening the thoracic spine (the middle and upper back), which is often stiff. This can improve breathing and relieve respiratory ailments.

Boosts Mood and Energy: As a backbend, Camel Pose is known for its ability to energize the body and uplift the mood. It stimulates the nervous system and can help alleviate mild depression and fatigue.

Improves Posture: By strengthening the back muscles and stretching the front of the body, Camel Pose helps in improving overall posture.

Therapeutic for Anxiety and Stress: The pose's opening effect on the chest and breathing can help relieve anxiety and stress, promoting a sense of well-being.

Promotes Confidence: Backbends like Camel Pose can also help open up the heart center, which is associated with vulnerability and openness, fostering a sense of courage and confidence.

Day 5
Vishuddha, or the Throat Chakra
Its element is Ether (Space)

Located at the throat area, Vishuddha governs the mouth, throat, thyroid, and parathyroid glands.
signifying its role in self-expression and communication.

Signs of a Balanced Vishuddha Chakra:
Clear and articulate communication
The ability to listen and understand others
Creative expression through speech, writing, or other forms
Honesty and truthfulness
Good sense of timing and rhythm in speech

Signs of an Imbalance:
Difficulty expressing thoughts or feelings
Fear of speaking or excessive shyness
Speaking too much or inappropriately
Stubbornness or holding onto old ways of thinking
Throat-related health issues, such as sore throats, thyroid problems, or dental issues

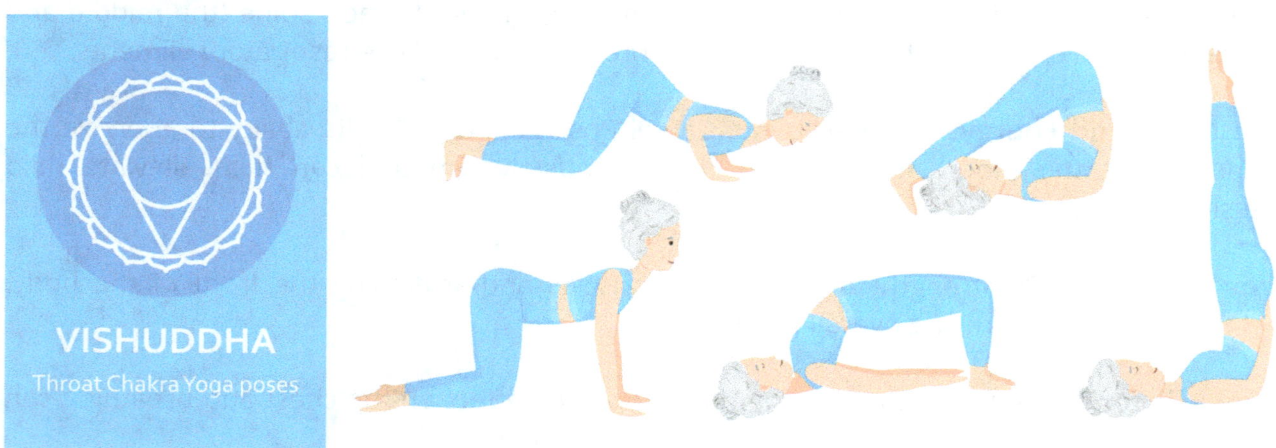

Pranayama:
Breathing exercises like Ujjayi Pranayama, also known as the Ocean Breath, can be particularly effective in stimulating the Throat Chakra.

Meditation and Mantras:
Meditating on the color blue or visualizing a blue light at the throat can help activate Vishuddha. Chanting the seed mantra "Ham" or singing can also be beneficial.

Affirmations:
Using affirmations that reinforce self-expression and communication, such as "I speak my truth freely and openly" or "I express myself with clarity and confidence," can support the balance of the Throat Chakra.

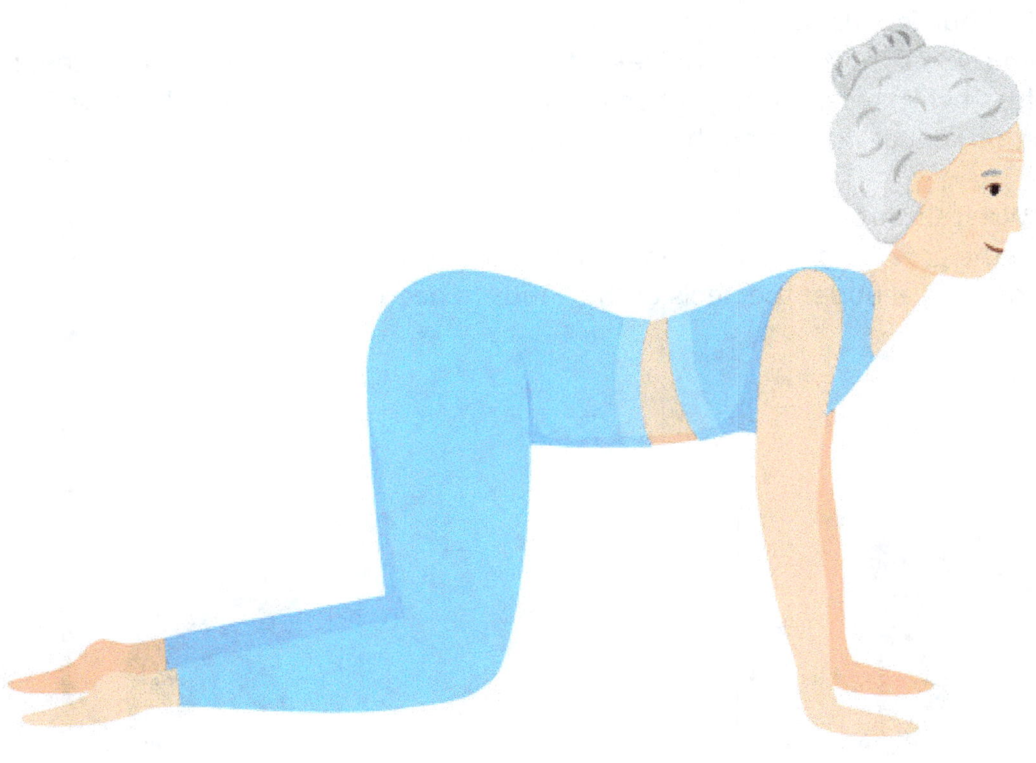

Standard Instructions:
Start on Hands and Knees: Position yourself on a yoga mat or padded surface, with your knees hip-width apart and your hands directly under your shoulders.

Cow Pose (Bitilasana): As you inhale, lower your belly towards the mat, lift your chin and chest, and gaze upwards. Allow your back to gently curve.

Cat Pose (Marjaryasana): As you exhale, round your spine toward the ceiling, tuck your chin towards your chest, and draw your belly in. Repeat the sequence for several breaths.

Use a Chair:
Sit in a chair with your feet flat on the floor and your spine long.
Perform the same spinal movements: Inhale and arch your back slightly, lifting your chest and gaze upwards for Cow. Exhale, round your spine, and drop your chin to your chest for Cat.
This seated version reduces stress on the wrists and knees.

Use Props for Wrist Comfort:
If performing on the ground, place a folded blanket under the knees for cushioning and use yoga wedges or a folded towel under the heels of the hands to decrease wrist extension.

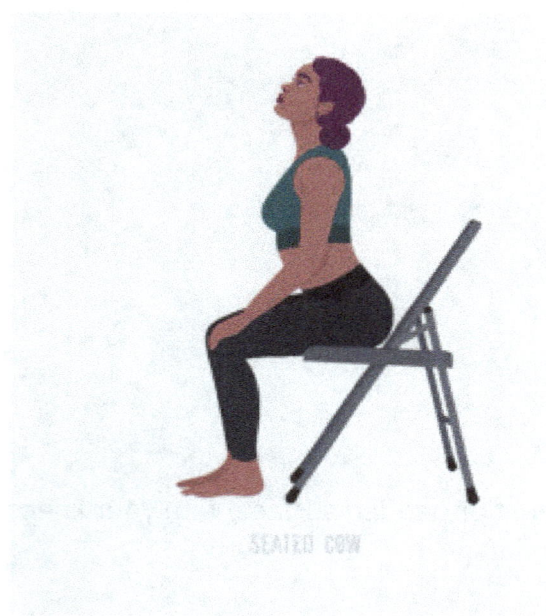

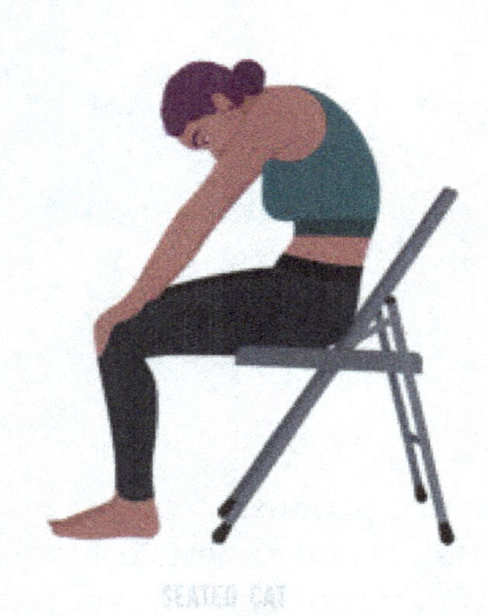

Benefits of Cat-Cow Pose:

Physical Benefits:

Increases Spinal Flexibility: The alternating movement between Cat and Cow poses helps improve the spine's flexibility and mobility. This gentle flexing and extending motion lubricates the spinal joints and can help prevent back stiffness and pain.

Strengthens and Stretches the Neck and Shoulders: The movement also involves the neck and shoulder muscles, providing a stretch that can relieve tension and enhance these areas.

Tones the Abdomen: In the Cat phase of the pose, the abdominal muscles are engaged as the spine rounds up, which can help tone and strengthen the core muscles.

Improves Posture: Regular practice of Cat-Cow helps improve spinal alignment and strengthen the muscles that support good posture.

Stimulates the Organs: The abdominal compression in the Cat Pose and the extension in the Cow Pose stimulate the internal organs, which can help improve digestive health and encourage detoxification.

Mental Benefits:

Reduces Stress and Calms the Mind: Cat-Cow's rhythmic, flowing movement helps calm the mind and can be meditative, reducing stress and mental fatigue.

Enhances Focus and Coordination: The coordination required to align the movements with the breath helps improve focus and mental clarity.

Therapeutic Benefits:

Relieves Lower Back Pain: The gentle stretching in Cat-Cow can be particularly beneficial for easing lower back pain, mainly if it's caused by tension or poor postural habits.

Increases Circulation: The movement helps improve blood circulation, especially around the spine and abdominal organs, promoting healing and overall health.

Beneficial During Pregnancy: For pregnant women, Cat-Cow can be a safe exercise for maintaining back health and managing stress during pregnancy, though modifications might be necessary as the pregnancy progresses.

Practice Tips:

Please perform this sequence on a yoga mat or another comfortable surface to protect your knees.

Always move within the comfort range and avoid over-extending, which could strain the back or neck.

Overall, Cat-Cow Pose offers a gentle yet effective way to enhance physical and mental well-being, making it ideal for yoga practitioners of all levels, from beginners to advanced.

Ashtanga Namaskara Asana
– Eight-Limbed Pose

To revisit the instructions for this pose, please refer to page 38

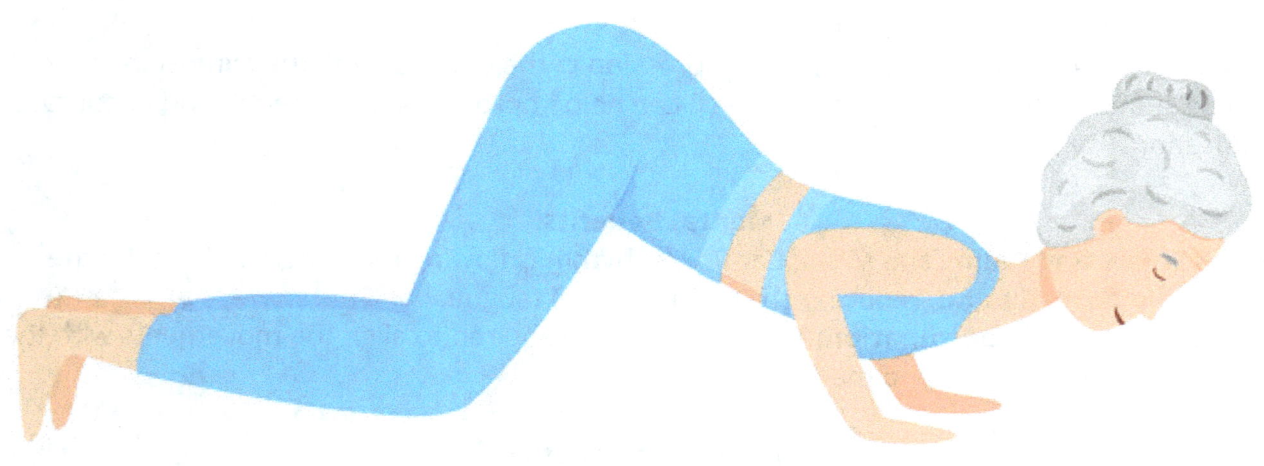

Bridge Pose (Setu Bandhasana)

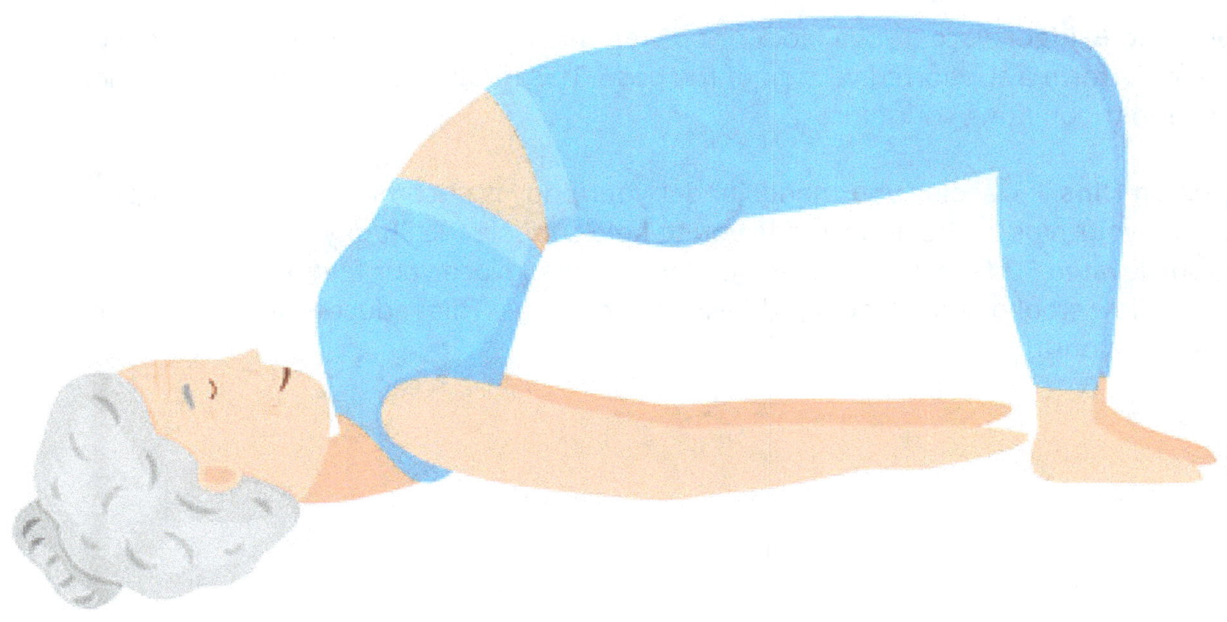

Start Position: Lie on your back with your knees bent and feet flat on the floor, hip-width apart. Place your arms alongside your body, palms facing down.

Lift Your Hips: Press your feet and arms firmly into the floor. Inhale, then lift your hips towards the ceiling, squeezing your buttocks and thighs. Keep your feet parallel to each other.

Shoulder Support: Clasp your hands under your lifted back and wiggle your shoulder blades closer together to open up your chest more. Keep your neck relaxed and your gaze upwards.

Hold and Breathe: Hold the pose for 4-8 breaths, focusing on lifting your hips higher with each inhalation and maintaining a firm foundation through your feet and shoulders.

To Release: Unclasp your hands and slowly lower your spine back to the floor, vertebra by vertebra, starting from the upper back to the lower back. Hug your knees to your chest for a gentle release.

Supported Bridge: Place a yoga block or bolster under your sacrum (the flat part of your lower back) to perform a supported version of the pose. This modification lets you experience the pose's benefits without lifting your hips.

Hands-on Hips: If clasping your hands under your body is uncomfortable, you can place your palms on your hips or the floor beside you to help support the lift of your pelvis.
Feet on Elevated Surface: For an even gentler variation, place your feet on an elevated surface, such as a low stool or a thick book, while lifting your hips. This reduces the angle of the lift, making it easier on your back.

Bridge Pose Benefits

Physical Benefits:

Strengthens the Back Muscles: Regular practice of Bridge Pose helps strengthen the lower back muscles and improves spinal alignment, which can alleviate and prevent back pain.

Opens the Chest and Shoulders: The pose lifts the chest, which helps open up the shoulders and chest, counteracting the effects of prolonged sitting or poor posture habits related to hunching over computers and phones.

Enhances Core Stability: By lifting the hips and engaging the abdominal muscles, Bridge Pose helps strengthen the core, which supports overall body alignment and balance.

Improves Digestion: The compression of the abdomen in Bridge Pose can help stimulate abdominal organs, improving digestion and relieving constipation.

Stimulates Thyroid and Lungs: The throat region is slightly compressed in this pose, which can help stimulate the thyroid gland. Additionally, the chest expansion helps increase lung capacity and improves respiratory function.

Mental Benefits:

Reduces Stress and Anxiety: The pose has a calming effect on the brain and can help alleviate stress and mild depression. This is mainly due to the chest opening, associated with improved respiratory capacity and enhanced relaxation.

Boosts Energy: As a mild inversion (with the heart lifted above the head), Bridge Pose can help increase circulation and energize the body and mind, especially during fatigue.

Improves Mood: By increasing circulation to the brain and stimulating the endocrine system, practicing Bridge Pose can help improve mood and increase feelings of well-being.

Plow Pose (Halasana)

Start Position: Lie on your back with your arms by your sides, palms facing down. Keep your legs extended and together.

Lift Your Legs: Inhale and use your abdominal muscles to lift your legs and hips off the floor, bringing your legs over your head towards the floor behind you. Keep your legs straight and toes pointed.

Support Your Back: Place your hands on your lower back, keeping your elbows close to each other on the floor.

Leg Position: If your toes touch the floor behind you, extend your legs, keeping them straight. Keep your hands on your back for support if your toes don't reach the floor.

Hold and Breathe: Stay in the pose for 5-10 breaths. Keep your neck and shoulders relaxed, and avoid turning your head to the side.

To Release: Support your back with your hands as you gently roll your spine back onto the floor, vertebra by vertebra, and lower your legs.

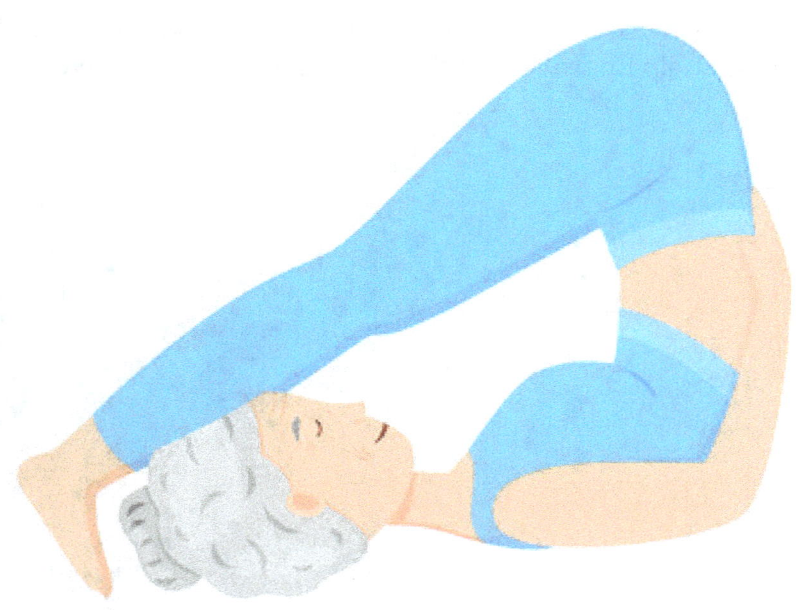

Use a Chair: Place a chair behind your head where your feet can land on the seat for support instead of reaching the floor. This reduces the strain on your back and neck.

Elevated Surface for Feet: If a chair is too low, rest your feet on an elevated platform, a stack of firm cushions, or yoga blocks.

Blanket Under Shoulders: Use a folded blanket under your shoulders to elevate your upper body slightly, reducing pressure on the neck and ensuring safer alignment.

Legs on Wall Variation: Instead of taking your legs over your head, stand your legs up the wall sideways and gently lower your back to the floor, bringing your hips closer to the wall. This variation simulates the inverted nature of Halasana without the intense spine flexion.

Plow Pose Benefits

Physical Benefits:

Stretches the Spine: Halasana provides a deep stretch to the spine's muscles, which can help relieve tension and promote spinal flexibility.

Strengthens the Shoulders and Neck: Supporting the body with the shoulders and arms strengthens these areas and can help improve posture.

Stimulates Thyroid and Parathyroid Glands: The neck position in Halasana helps stimulate the thyroid and parathyroid glands, which regulate metabolism and calcium levels.

Enhances Digestion: The folding of the abdomen compresses the internal organs, which can help stimulate digestion and relieve constipation.

Improves Circulation: As an inversion, Halasana helps reverse the blood flow, improving circulation and energizing the body.

Mental Benefits:

Reduces Stress and Fatigue: Inversion can soothe the nervous system, reducing stress and alleviating fatigue.

Promotes Mental Calmness: The pose requires focus and balance, which can help calm the mind and reduce anxiety.

Therapeutic Benefits:

Menopause and Menstruation: Halasana can help ease symptoms associated with menopause and, when practiced regularly, may also benefit women during menstruation by promoting relaxation.

Insomnia: Halasana can improve sleep patterns and help combat insomnia by promoting physical and mental relaxation.

Backache: Regular practice can strengthen the back muscles and alleviate discomfort, helping to manage chronic back pain.

Caution:

While Halasana is beneficial, it's only suitable for some. People with neck issues, high blood pressure, or glaucoma should avoid this pose or practice it only under the guidance of a knowledgeable instructor. Beginners should start gently and gradually increase the intensity to avoid overstraining the neck or back.

Shoulder Stand (Sarvangasana)

Start Position: Begin by lying flat on your back with your legs and arms by your sides, palms facing down.

Lift Legs: Press your arms and hands onto the floor to lift your legs and hips toward the ceiling. Use your hands to support your lower back, keeping your elbows close to each other.

Align Your Body: Straighten your legs and align them over your hips so your body forms a straight line from the shoulders to the feet. Focus on lifting through the balls of your feet to keep the legs active.

Hold and Breathe: Keep your chin tucked into your chest, with your neck long. Hold the pose for 5-10 breaths, aiming for a steady and smooth breath.

To Release: Slowly lower your legs over your head into Plow Pose (Halasana) as a transition, then gently roll your spine back down to the floor, vertebra by vertebra. Please rest on your back for a few minutes before you move.

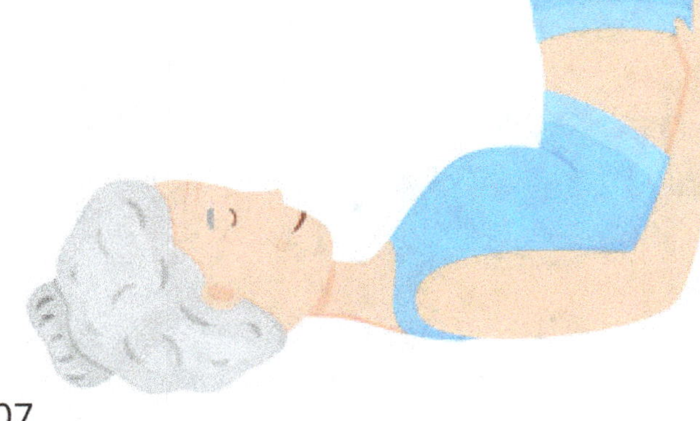

Use a Wall: Start with your feet flat against a wall with your hips close to the base of the wall. Lift into the pose by pushing your feet against the wall to help lift your hips, then walk your feet up the wall as you lift higher.

Chair Support: Place a chair near your head so when you lift your legs up, you can rest them on the seat of the chair instead of lifting them straight into the air. This reduces the strain on the neck and shoulders.

Stacked Pillows or Bolsters: Use stacked pillows or bolsters under your shoulders to elevate them. This decreases the angle between the neck and the torso, reducing pressure on the cervical spine.

Legs on Chair: For an even gentler inversion, lie on your back with your lower legs resting on the seat of a chair. This inverted position allows you to experience some of the benefits of Shoulder Stand without the full inversion.

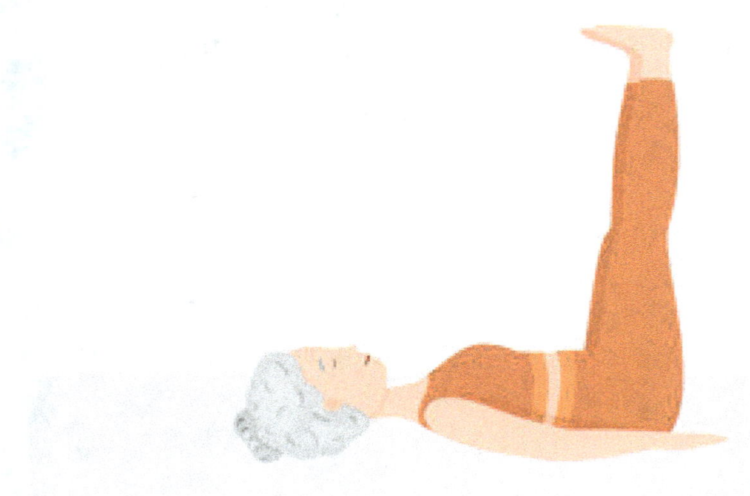

Legs Up the Wall Pose
Viparita Karani

Benefits of practicing Shoulder Stand:

Physical Benefits:
Stimulates the Thyroid and Parathyroid Glands: The chin lock (Jalandhara Bandha) created in this pose helps stimulate the thyroid glands, regulate metabolism, and improve the health of the endocrine system.
Enhances Circulation: As an inversion, Shoulder Stand increases blood flow to the brain, which can help improve mental function and vitality. It also enhances venous return and can improve cardiovascular health.
Strengthens the Upper Body: The shoulders, arms, and upper back must stabilize the body, maintaining these areas.
Improves Digestive Function: The change in gravity affects the abdominal organs, including the digestive tract, which can help alleviate constipation and promote better digestion.
Boosts Immunity: The improved circulation and stimulation of the thyroid and lymph nodes can enhance immune system functionality.

Mental Benefits:
Reduces Stress and Mild Depression: The inverted nature of the pose has a calming effect on the brain, helping to reduce anxiety, stress, and mild depression.
Improves Focus and Concentration: Maintaining balance and alignment in the Shoulder Stand requires focus and mental clarity, which can translate into enhanced concentration outside yoga practice.

Therapeutic Benefits:
Relieves Symptoms of Menopause: Shoulder Stand can help alleviate some symptoms of menopause through its regulating effects on the thyroid and endocrine system.
Beneficial for Insomnia: The calming effect on the nervous system can promote better sleep patterns and help combat insomnia.
Supports Sinus Health: The inversion aids in draining mucus from the lungs and nasal passages, which can benefit people suffering from sinusitis.

Caution:
Shoulder Stand is a complex and advanced yoga pose that should be cautiously approached, especially by beginners or those with known health issues such as high blood pressure, heart conditions, neck problems, or during menstruation. You can always practice under the guidance of a knowledgeable instructor and consider using supportive props or modifications, such as performing the pose against a wall or with blankets under the shoulders to reduce strain on the neck.

Overall, Sarvangasana is a highly beneficial pose that impacts health's physical, mental, and therapeutic aspects, making it a valuable addition to a regular yoga practice.

Day 6
Ajna, the Third Eye Chakra
Element: Light

Located in the forehead, between the eyebrows, it is often associated with the pineal gland. It is considered the center of intuition, foresight, and inner wisdom

Signs of a Balanced Ajna Chakra:

Strong intuition and a sense of inner knowing
Ability to see beyond deceit and illusions
Mental clarity and focused decision-making
Openness to inspiration and imaginative thought
Spiritual awareness and connection to the universe

Signs of an Imbalance:

Confusion or indecision
Feeling stuck in the daily grind without a sense of purpose
Over-reliance on rationality or, conversely, being caught up in fantasies
Headaches, blurred vision, or eye strain
Insomnia or nightmares

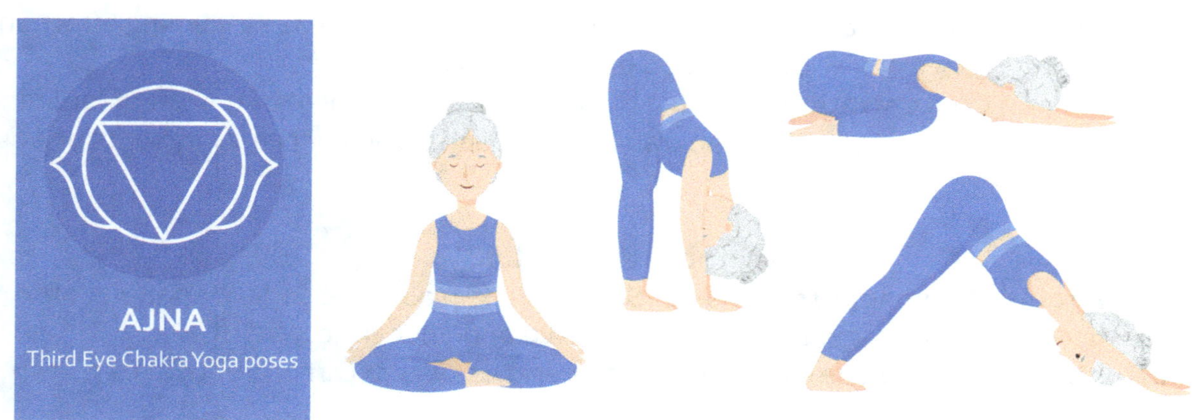

Mindfulness Affirmations for Ajna Chakra:
"I trust my intuition and always allow it to guide me."
"My inner vision is clear and strong."

Mindfulness Meditation:
Focusing your meditation on the space between the eyebrows can help activate Ajna. Visualizing an indigo light or flame in this area is particularly effective.

Mindful Breathing_Pranayama:
Pay attention to your breath, noticing how it feels as you inhale and exhale. This practice can help quiet the mind, making it easier to hear your inner voice and intuition.
Alternate nostril breathing (Nadi Shodhana) is beneficial for this purpose.

Hasta Padasana - Standing Forward Bend

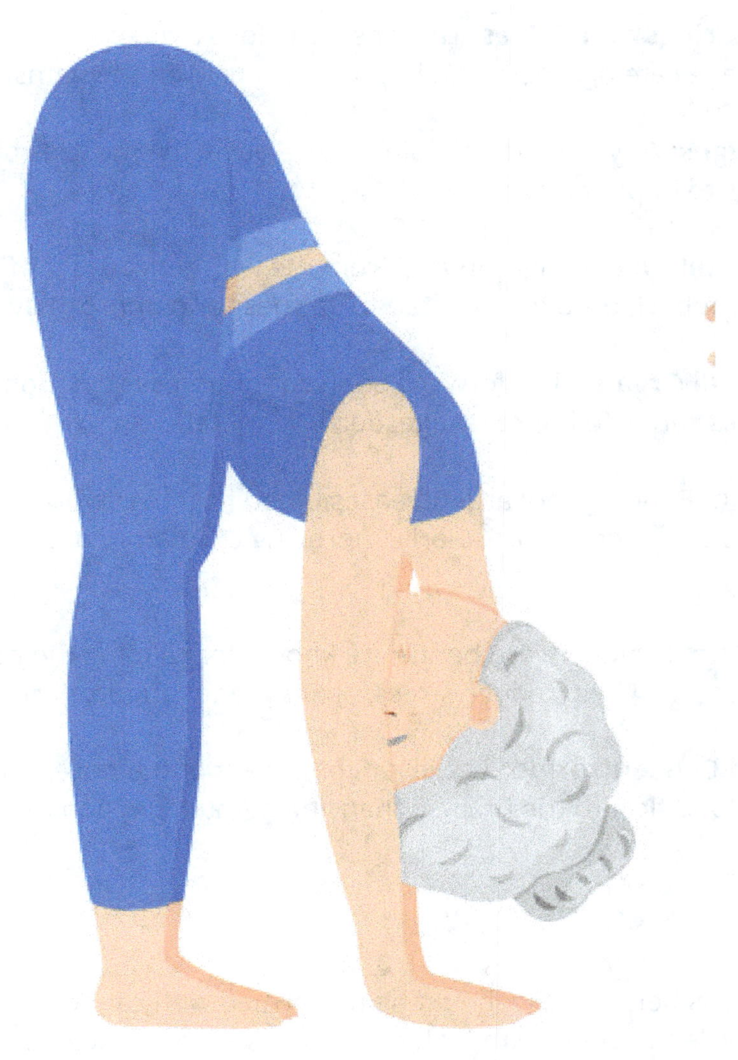

Advantages of practicing Hasta Padasana:

Physical Benefits:
Stretches the Hamstrings and Calves: This pose provides a deep stretch to the back of the legs, which can help alleviate tightness and improve flexibility in the hamstrings and calves.

Strengthens the Thighs: As you work to maintain the pose, the muscles of the thighs are engaged, which helps to improve them.

Improves Spine Flexibility: Bending forward from the waist encourages flexibility in the spine, which can help prevent back problems related to stiffness and improve overall spinal health.

Stimulates Abdominal Organs: The forward bend compresses the abdominal area, stimulating the organs within. This can help improve digestion and metabolism.

Enhances Circulation: Bending forward increases blood flow to the brain, which can invigorate and rejuvenate the body systems, particularly improving circulatory health.

Mental Benefits:
Reduces Stress and Anxiety: Forward bends are known for calming the mind and nervous system. Hasta Padasana can help reduce stress, anxiety, and fatigue, promoting inner peace.

Improves Focus and Concentration: The inversion aspect of the pose, with the head below the heart, can increase blood flow to the brain, enhancing mental functions like focus and concentration.

Caution:
While Hasta Padasana is beneficial, it should be performed with caution by those with back injuries or spinal disorders. People with high blood pressure or glaucoma might also need to avoid complete forward bends or practice a modified version of the pose under the guidance of a qualified instructor.

This pose is highly valued in yoga for its ability to promote physical and mental wellness through its simple yet profound practice.

Adho Mukha Svanasana – Downward-Facing Dog Pose

To revisit the instructions for this pose,
please refer to page 33

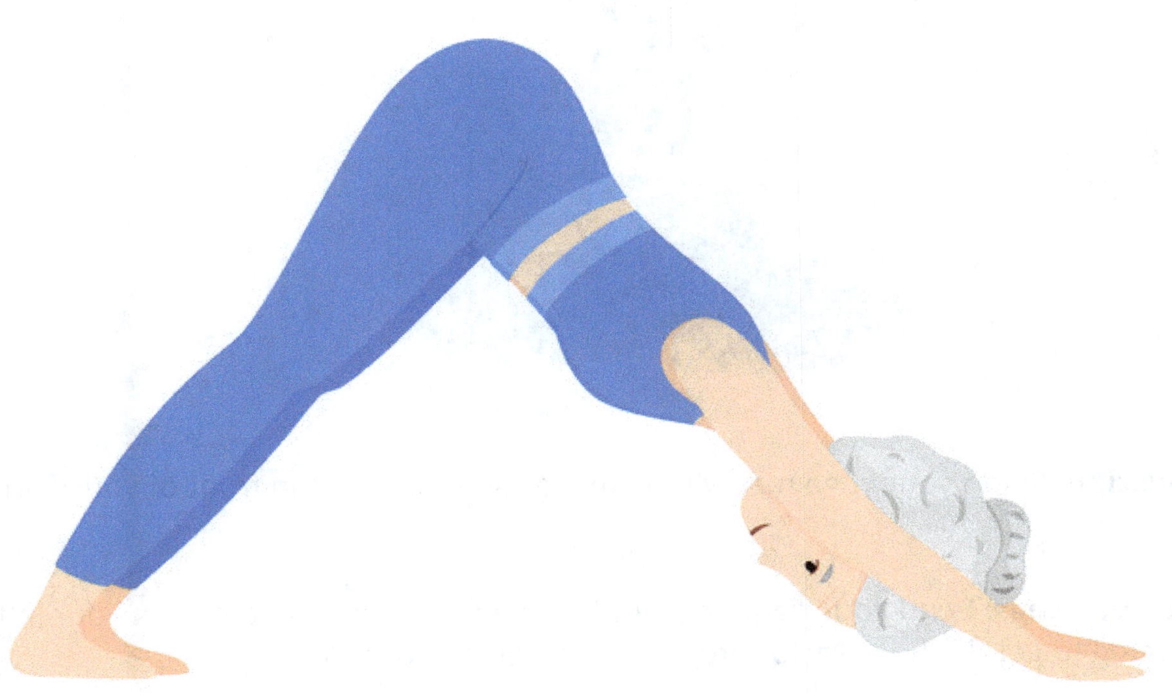

Lotus Pose (Padmasana)

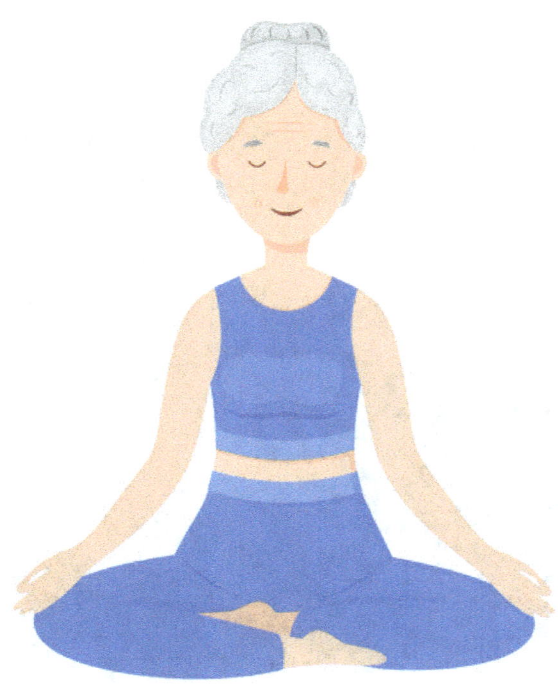

Start Position: Sit on your yoga mat with your legs stretched out in front of you, spine straight.

Prepare Your Legs: Bend your right knee and gently place your right foot on your left thigh, aiming to get the heel as close to the abdomen as possible.

Position the Other Leg: Repeat with your left leg, placing your left foot on your right thigh. Ensure both knees are touching the floor, and the soles of your feet are pointing upward.

Spine Alignment: Keep your spine erect, and place your hands on your knees in a mudra (gesture) of your choice, commonly with palms facing up.

Hold and Breathe: Maintain the pose while taking deep, even breaths. Focus on relaxing your hips and gently pushing your knees towards the floor.

To Release: Carefully reverse the legs' position, one at a time, returning to a seated position with your legs stretched out.

Modification for Seniors

Half Lotus (Ardha Padmasana): If full Lotus is too intense, try placing only one foot on the opposite thigh, keeping the other beneath the opposite knee. Switch legs to balance the stretch on both sides.

Use Props: Sit on a folded blanket or cushion to elevate your hips and ease pressure on your knees. This adjustment helps tilt your pelvis forward, aiding in hip opening.

Supported Knees: Place cushions or folded blankets under each knee if your knees don't comfortably reach the floor. This helps reduce strain on the hip joints and knees.

Seated on a Chair: Sit on a chair and cross your legs at the ankles for a gentler variation. This variation allows you to work on hip opening without the strain of the whole or half-lotus positions.

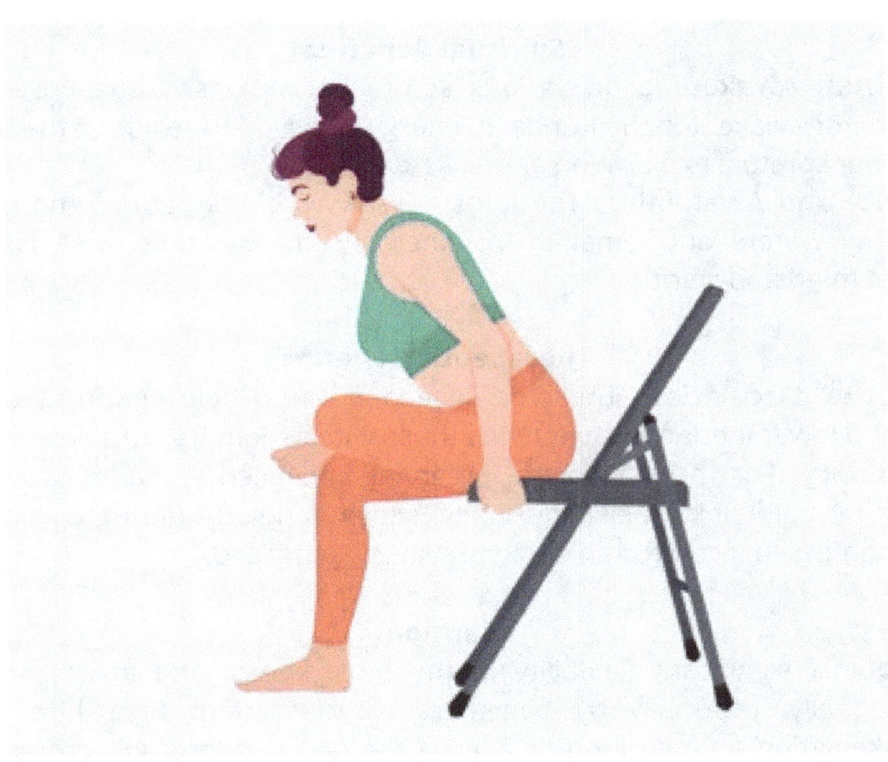

Benefits of Lotus Pose

Physical Benefits:

Improves Flexibility: Regular practice of Padmasana gradually increases flexibility in the hips, knees, and ankles. This can be particularly beneficial for those who sit for long periods or have stiff lower bodies.

Stabilizes the Pelvis: By positioning the legs in a locked arrangement, Padmasana helps stabilize the pelvis, which can lead to improved posture and spine alignment during seated meditation.

Stimulates Abdominal Organs: The seated position of Lotus Pose puts gentle pressure on the lower abdomen, stimulating the abdominal organs and aiding in digestion and the function of reproductive organs.

Mental Benefits:

Promotes Calm and Focus: Lotus Pose is traditionally used for meditation because its naturally balanced and symmetrical posture promotes physical stability and helps cultivate mental calm and focus.

Reduces Stress: Padmasana facilitates deep breathing and meditation, helping reduce stress and anxiety and promoting a sense of grounding and inner peace.

Spiritual Benefits:

Enhances Spiritual Awakening: In various spiritual traditions, Lotus Pose is considered a powerful posture for awakening the Kundalini energy, believed to reside at the base of the spine. It facilitates deeper spiritual exploration and enlightenment.

Symbol of Purity and Awakening: The lotus flower symbolizes purity and detachment, as it blooms in muddy waters but remains unstained. Practicing Lotus Pose is a metaphor for transforming the mind and spirit.

Therapeutic Benefits:

Encourages Better Circulation: The cross-legged position helps improve circulation in the lumbar region and lower limbs, which benefits those with sedentary lifestyles.

Supports Pregnancy: For those who are pregnant and used to Padmasana, continuing the practice can aid in maintaining pelvis flexibility, which is helpful during childbirth. However, it should only be continued if comfortable and previously practiced.

Caution:

Padmasana requires significant flexibility in the hips, knees, and ankles, and it should be approached gradually, especially by beginners or those with tight hips or knee issues. Modifications, like sitting on a cushion or placing the feet less intensely crossed, can make the pose accessible while reducing the risk of injury.

Overall, Padmasana offers a range of benefits, supporting physical health and aiding in mental focus and spiritual development when integrated into a regular practice.

Child's Pose (Balasana)

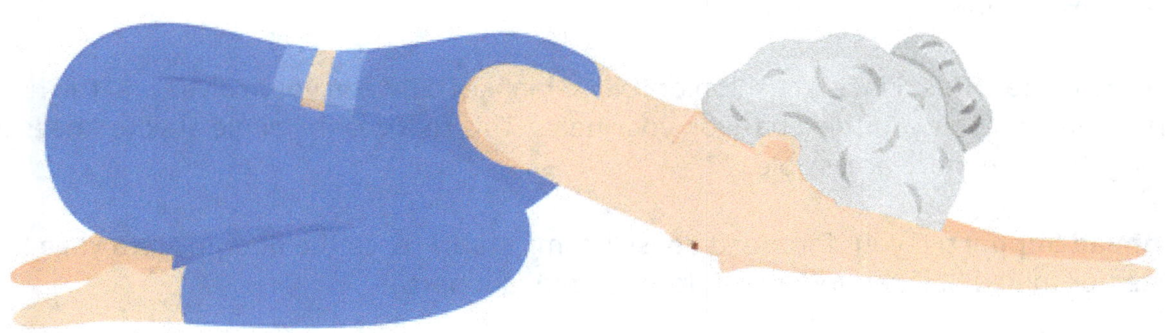

Start Position:
Begin on your hands and knees on the mat, knees hip-width apart, toes touching.

Sit Back: Exhale and lower your hips towards your heels, sitting back as far as comfortable.

Extend Arms: Stretch your arms out in front of you on the mat, palms facing down, or let your arms rest alongside your body, palms facing up, towards your feet.

Rest Your Forehead: Gently lower your forehead to the mat. If your forehead doesn't reach the mat, use a folded blanket or pillow for support.

Hold and Breathe: Breathe deeply while relaxing your spine, shoulders, and arms. Hold the pose for as long as it's comfortable, focusing on a deep, relaxing breath.

To Release: Use your hands to push yourself back up to a seated position on your heels, then transition to hands and knees.

Knees Apart: If sitting back on your heels is uncomfortable, widen your knees further apart while keeping your big toes touching. This creates more space for your torso and can relieve discomfort in your hips or knees.

Support Under Hips: Place a cushion or folded blanket between your calves and thighs if you can't comfortably sit your hips back on your heels. This reduces the angle at your knees and hips, making the pose more accessible.

Forehead Support: If your forehead doesn't comfortably reach the floor, place a yoga block, bolster, or folded blanket under your forehead for support.

Arms by Your Side: If extending your arms forward is uncomfortable, let your arms rest alongside your body with your hands near your feet. This can reduce tension in your shoulders and neck.

Child's Pose Benefits

Physical Benefits:
Releases Tension in the Back and Shoulders: Balasana stretches and relaxes the spine, shoulders, and neck, which helps to relieve tension and pain in these areas. This gentle stretch can be particularly beneficial after long periods of sitting or standing.

Stretches the Hips, Thighs, and Ankles: The pose involves sitting back on the heels and folding forward, stretching the hips, thighs, and ankles. This can help alleviate stiffness and improve flexibility in these areas.

Promotes Flexibility in the Spine: The forward bend in the Child's Pose helps elongate and align the spine, improving overall spinal flexibility and health.

Aids in Digestion: The forward fold compresses the abdomen, stimulating digestion and alleviating bloating and constipation.

Mental Benefits:
Calms the Mind: The pose encourages deep breathing, which has a natural calming effect on the nervous system. This can help reduce stress, anxiety, and mental fatigue.

Encourages Relaxation and Rejuvenation: Balasana is often used as a pose of surrender, allowing for moments of rest and recuperation during yoga practice. This can help rejuvenate the mind and body, particularly during strenuous sessions.

Improves Focus and Concentration: The child's pose fosters a state of calm and introspection, helping clear the mind and improve focus and concentration once you resume activity.

Therapeutic Benefits:
Relieves Headaches: Child's Pose can help alleviate tension headaches by promoting relaxation and reducing stress.

Reduces Fatigue: As a restful pose, Balasana can help lower fatigue levels, especially if practiced with controlled breathing.

Helps in Managing Symptoms of Depression and Anxiety: The soothing effect of the pose on the nervous system can be beneficial in managing depression and anxiety, providing a sense of grounding and stability.

.Located at the top of the head or slightly above it, Sahasrara is the point of spiritual connection to the divine, the universe, or whatever higher power one believes in.

Signs of a Balanced :

A deep sense of peace and inner harmony
Feeling connected to a higher power and the universe
Experiencing unconditional love and oneness with all
Living in the present moment and having a sense of pure awareness
Displaying a high level of spiritual wisdom and insight

Signs of an Imbalance:

Spiritual cynicism or a lack of direction and purpose
Feeling disconnected or isolated from others and the world
Overwhelming fear of death or excessive attachment to material things
Lack of inspiration or closed-mindedness

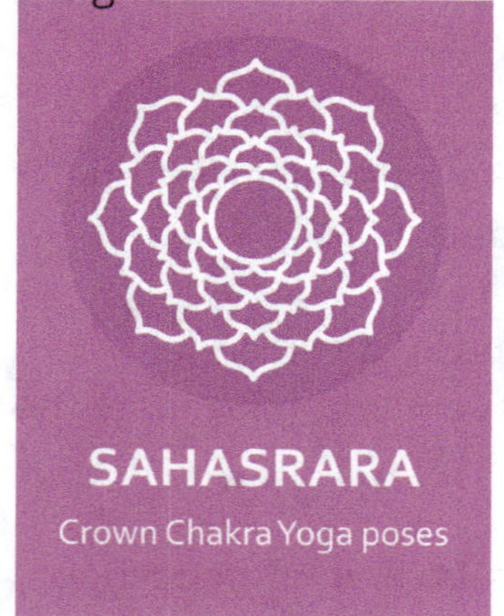

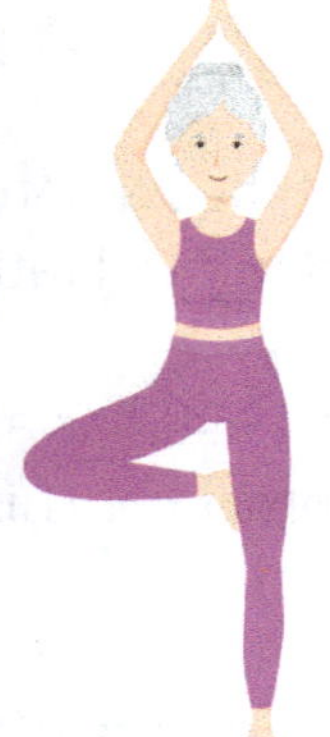
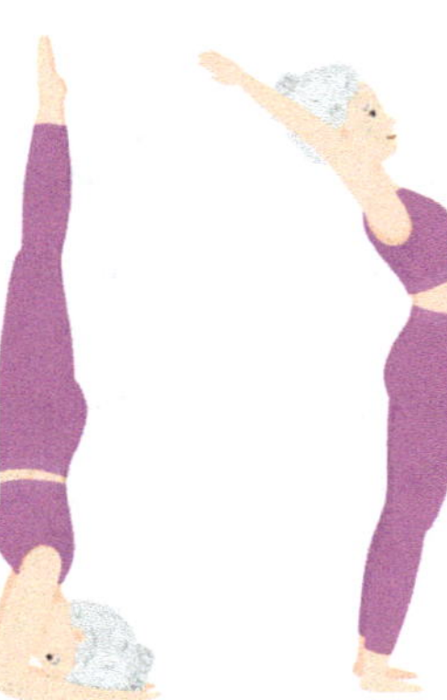
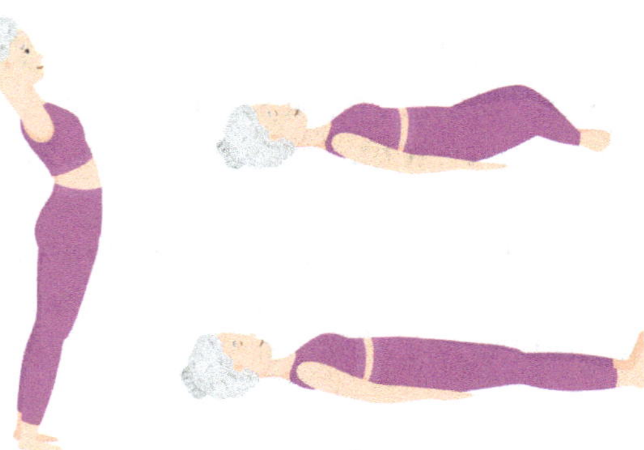

Affirmations:
"I am connected to the universal source of knowledge and wisdom."
"I am a vessel for light, love, and the divine energy of the universe."
"I understand the impermanence of physical existence and embrace the eternal spirit within me."

Mindfulness and Awareness Practices:
Cultivating awareness in every moment, practicing mindfulness, and observing your thoughts without attachment

Prayer and Devotion:
Engaging in prayer, devotion, or any practice that helps you connect with a sense of something greater than yourself can help balance Sahasrara.

Hasta Uttanasana - Raised Arms Pose

**To revisit the instructions for this pose,
please refer to page 27**

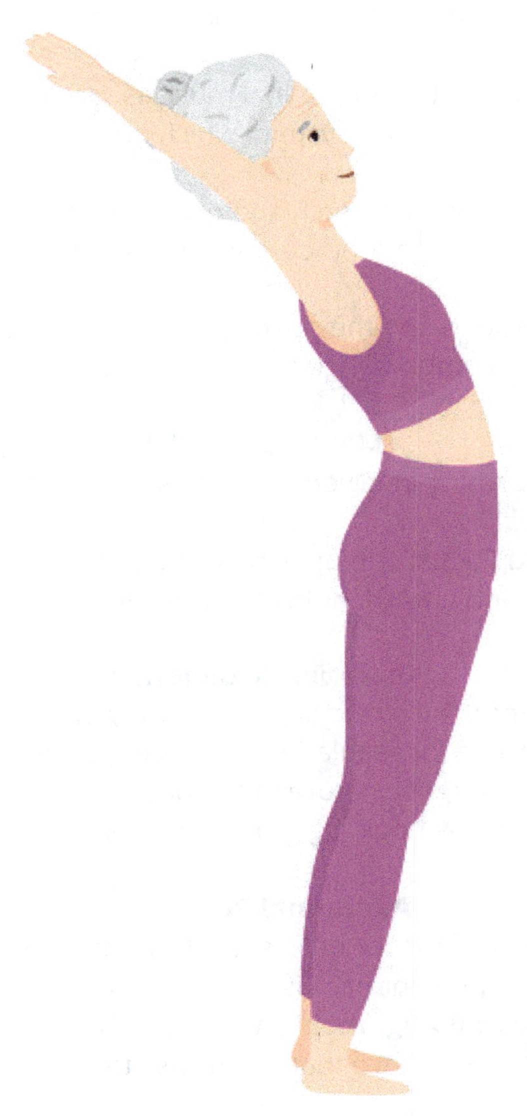

Benefits of Raised Arms Pose

Physical Benefits:
Stretches and Tones the Muscles: This pose stretches the abdomen, chest, and shoulders while toning the arms and spine. Regular practice can enhance flexibility in these areas and improve posture.
Improves Digestion: By stretching the abdominal muscles, Hasta Uttanasana stimulates the abdominal organs, including the digestive system, which can help to improve digestion and relieve constipation.
Increases Lung Capacity: The upward stretch and backbend open up the chest, allowing for deeper inhalations and exhalations. This increase in lung capacity can improve overall respiratory efficiency.
Energizes the Body: The backbend and the opening of the chest help to invigorate the body and mind, making it a great pose to combat fatigue and provide a boost of energy.

Mental Benefits:
Reduces Stress: The deep breathing involved in this pose helps to calm the mind, reduce anxiety, and lower stress levels.
Enhances Concentration and Focus: The upward stretch encourages mental alertness and focus, as maintaining balance and alignment in the pose requires concentration.

Therapeutic Benefits:
Stimulates Endocrine Function: The stretching of the body in this pose can help stimulate the thyroid gland, which is responsible for regulating metabolic processes.
Aids in Mild Depression: The energetic nature of the pose and the opening of the chest can have a mild antidepressant effect by boosting mood and energy levels.

Additional Benefits:
Improves Spinal Health: Regular practice of Hasta Uttanasana can improve the flexibility and strength of the spine, helping to prevent back issues.
Promotes a Sense of Balance and Alignment: As you reach upwards and stretch the body, you cultivate a sense of alignment and balance that can translate into other physical activities and daily life.

Caution:
This pose involves a backbend, so it should be practiced with care, especially by those with back pain, spinal injuries, or high blood pressure. It is essential to engage the core to support the lower back during the pose, and modifications may be necessary depending on individual flexibility and strength.

Hasta Uttanasana offers a comprehensive range of benefits that enhance both physical health and mental well-being, making it a valuable addition to any yoga practice.

Tree Pose

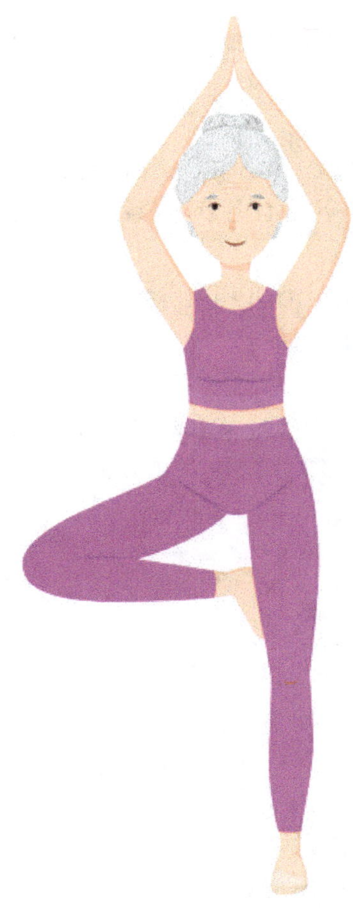

Begin in Mountain Pose: Stand tall, assemble your feet, and balance your weight evenly.

Place Your Foot: Shift weight to your left foot, and place your right foot on your inner left thigh, calf, or ankle, avoiding the knee.

Find Balance: Bring hands to the prayer position at your heart. Focus on a fixed point in front of you.

Open the Hip: Press your right knee back, aligning both hips forward.

Option to Extend Arms: If stable, reach arms overhead, palms facing or touching.

Hold for 5-10 Breaths: Maintain posture, breathing evenly.
Release and Repeat: Return to Mountain Pose and switch sides.

Modifications and Safety Tips:

Wall for Support: Stand near a wall for support if balancing is challenging. Place a hand on the wall until you feel stable.

Foot Placement: If placing your foot on your inner thigh is difficult, you can put it below the knee on the calf or ankle with the toes touching the ground for extra stability.

Focus on Alignment: Ensure your standing leg is straight but not locked at the knee, and keep your chest lifted and open.

Listen to Your Body: Respect your body's limitations. If you feel any pain or excessive strain, especially in the knee of your standing leg, adjust your foot placement or exit the pose.

Tree Pose Benefits

Physical Benefits:

Improves Balance and Stability: One of the primary benefits of Tree Pose is that it helps improve your sense of balance and stability, which is crucial for everyday activities and other physical pursuits.

Strengthens Legs: Standing on one leg strengthens the muscles of that leg, including the thighs, calves, ankles, and feet. The supporting leg's muscles become more toned and robust as they work to maintain balance.

Opens the Hips: By placing the foot of the non-standing leg on the inner thigh, calf, or ankle of the standing leg (never on the knee), the pose helps open the hips and improve hip flexibility.

Enhances Core Stability: To maintain balance in Tree Pose, the core must be engaged. This engagement strengthens the abdominal muscles and the lower back, supporting overall posture and body alignment.

Mental Benefits:

Improves Focus and Concentration: Balancing on one leg requires mental focus and concentration to maintain stability, which can help improve cognitive functions related to attention.

Reduces Stress: The concentration required in Tree Pose can help take your mind off daily stressors and instill a sense of calm and relaxation.

Therapeutic Benefits:

Sciatica Relief: Regular practice of Tree Pose can help alleviate discomfort from sciatica by strengthening the lower back and stretching the thighs.

Enhances Neurological Coordination: Balancing poses like Tree Pose help enhance neuromuscular coordination, promoting better coordination and proprioception (body position awareness).

Additional Benefits:

Promotes Self-confidence: Successfully maintaining balance in Tree Pose can boost self-confidence and body awareness.

Encourages Patience and Perseverance: Balancing poses require patience to master and maintain, which can translate into other areas of life, fostering a sense of perseverance.

Symbolic Meaning: In many traditions, the tree is a symbol of life and connectivity between the earth and the sky. Practicing Tree Pose can also be a meditative experience, reflecting personal growth and connection to one's environment.

Caution:

People with high blood pressure or current or recent knee injuries should modify or avoid this pose. Modifications can include performing the pose near a wall for support or placing the foot lower on the leg to reduce strain

Salamba Sirsasana, or Supported Headstand

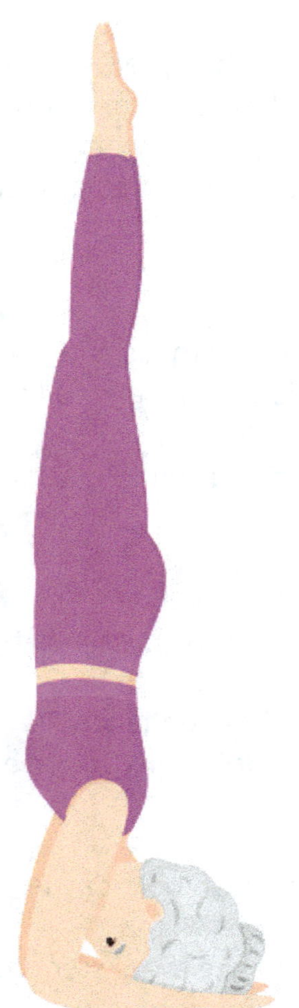

Preparation: Begin on your hands and knees on a yoga mat. Place a folded blanket or a firm cushion under your head for extra support.

Interlock Your Fingers: Interlock your fingers and place your forearms on the mat, creating a triangle base with your arms. Position Your Head: Place the crown of your head on the mat, cradled by your interlocked hands. Ensure your back is straight.

Lift Your Hips: Tuck your toes under, lift your hips, and straighten your legs like in Downward-Facing Dog. Walk your feet towards your head to shift the weight to your shoulders.

Raise Your Legs: One at a time, gently lift your feet off the ground, keeping your knees bent initially. With control, straighten your legs upwards. Your body should be in a straight line from head to toes.

Hold and Breathe: Maintain the pose for a few breaths, focusing on balance and stability.

To Come Out: Gently lower your legs back down the same way you entered the pose. Rest in Child's Pose for a few breaths.

Legs Up The Wall: Instead of performing the full inversion, seniors can practice "Legs Up The Wall" (Viparita Karani) as an alternative. This pose offers similar benefits, such as increased circulation and relaxation, without the risk associated with inversions.

Dolphin Pose: Practice Dolphin Pose to build shoulder and core strength as a preparatory exercise. It provides the foundation needed for a headstand without the risk of balancing the entire body weight on the head and neck.

Use a Wall: If attempting a supported headstand, practicing near a wall as a safety measure can help prevent falling and allow for gradual progression into the full pose.

Chair Support: Place a chair against the wall. Sit on the chair facing away from the wall and place your feet on the wall at hip height. Lean forward, placing your elbows on your knees, and interlock your fingers behind your head. This position mimics the upper body alignment of Salamba Sirsasana without the inversion.

Always prioritize safety and comfort, especially when practicing challenging poses like Salamba Sirsasana. It's highly recommended to practice under the guidance of a qualified yoga instructor.

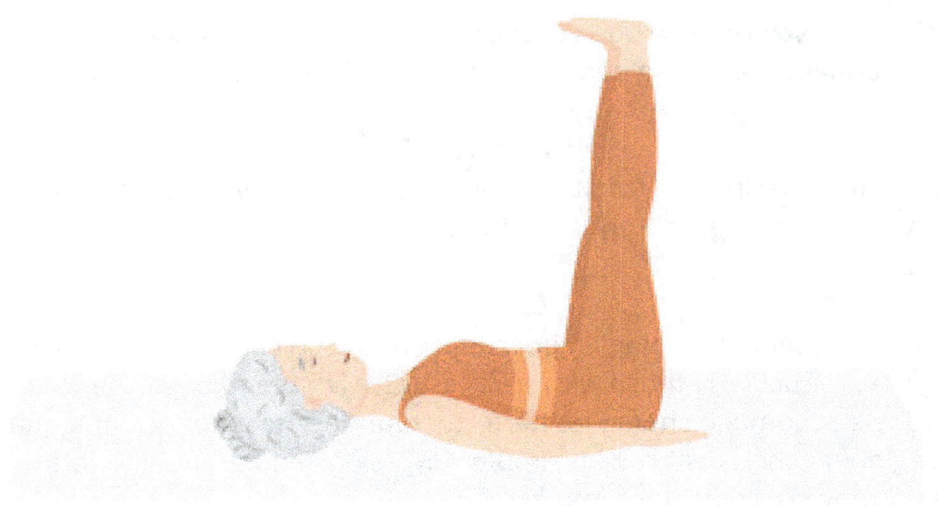

Legs Up the Wall Pose
Viparita Karani

Salamba Sirsasana Benefits

Physical Benefits:

Strengthens Upper Body: Sirsasana helps to maintain the shoulders, arms, and upper back, as these areas support most of the body's weight during the pose.

Improves Core Strength: Balancing in a headstand requires significant core engagement, which helps to strengthen core muscle strength, stability, and balance.

Enhances Circulation: As an inversion, Sirsasana reverses the expected effects of gravity on the body, improving blood flow to the brain, eyes, scalp, and facial skin. This increased circulation can help to refresh the circulatory and lymphatic systems.

Stimulates Endocrine Glands: The pose stimulates and helps regulate the activities of the pituitary and pineal glands in the brain, which are critical to the body's overall homeostasis and hormone production.

Mental Benefits:

Relieves Stress: The inverted position can have a calming effect on the brain, helping to relieve stress and decrease mild depression.

Improves Focus and Concentration: Maintaining balance in Sirsasana enhances focus and concentration. The increased blood flow to the brain also supports these mental functions.

Therapeutic Benefits:

Alleviates Symptoms of Menopause: Sirsasana can help manage the symptoms of menopause through improved endocrine function and stress reduction.

May Aid in Treating Insomnia: The calming effects of the pose can help improve sleep patterns and fight insomnia.

Helps in Sinusitis and Asthma: The pose encourages deeper breathing and can help clear sinus blockages while potentially benefiting people with asthma by improving lung capacity.

Spiritual Benefits:

Promotes Spiritual Insight: In yoga tradition, inversions are believed to increase prana (life force), aid in spiritual awakening, and enhance the practitioner's ability to maintain mental clarity and physical health.

Caution:

Despite its benefits, Sirsasana is a complex pose that should be cautiously approached. It's not suitable for everyone, particularly those with neck issues, high blood pressure, heart conditions, or eye problems like glaucoma. It should be performed under the guidance of a qualified yoga instructor, and beginners should start with simpler inversions and gradually work up to Sirsasana as their strength and balance improve.

Reclining Butterfly Pose (Supta Baddha Konasana)

Start Position:
Begin by lying on your back on a yoga mat or a comfortable surface. Ensure your spine is straight, and your arms rest comfortably at your sides, palms facing up.

Feet Together: Bend your knees and bring the soles of your feet together, letting your knees fall open to the sides, creating a diamond shape with your legs.

Adjust Your Position: Gently shift your pelvis and spine to ensure no discomfort in your lower back. Your tailbone should extend towards your heels to elongate the lower back.

Relax into the Pose: Allow your knees to fall towards the floor naturally. Avoid forcing them down, as the goal is to relax into the stretch without straining the hip joints or inner thighs.

Arms and Hands: Your arms can remain at your sides, or you can place one hand on your heart and one on your abdomen to connect more deeply with your breath and body.

Hold and Breathe: Stay in this pose for 5-10 minutes, focusing on deep, slow breaths that expand your abdomen and chest. With each exhale, imagine any tension in your hips and groin melting away.

To Release: Use your hands to support your knees as you bring them together gently. Roll onto one side in the fetal position before using your hands to press yourself up to a seated position.

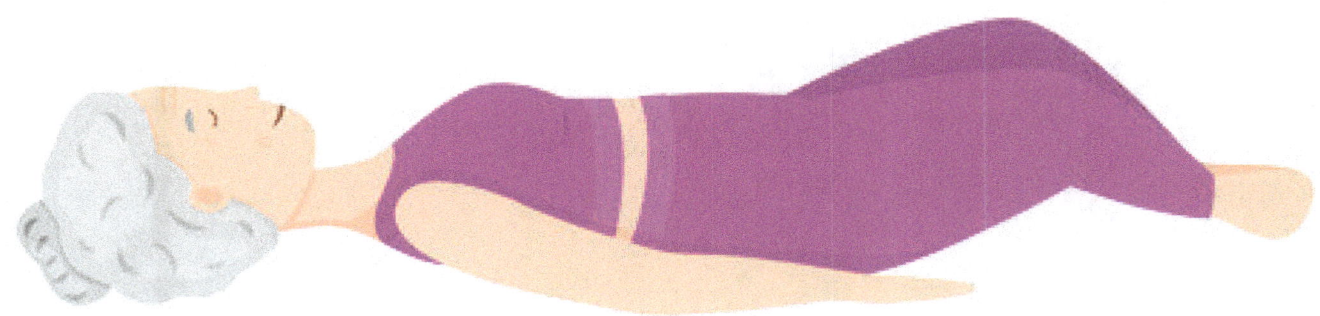

Modifications for Comfort and Support:

Support Under Knees: Place folded blankets, bolsters, or yoga blocks under each knee or thigh for support. This helps reduce the intensity of the hip opener and allows your muscles to relax more fully.

Under the Back: To provide additional lower back support or ease discomfort, slide a bolster or folded blanket under your spine, from the lower back to the head.

Eye Pillow: Place a weighted eye pillow over your eyes to help deepen relaxation and block out distracting light.

Physical Benefits:

Improves Hip Flexibility: Butterfly Pose is excellent for opening the hips and increasing the range of motion in the hip joints. This is particularly beneficial for those who sit for long periods or have tight hips.

Stretches the Groin and Inner Thighs: The pose provides a deep stretch to the muscles of the inner thighs and groin, which can help alleviate tightness and improve leg flexibility.

Stimulates Abdominal Organs: The forward bending movement in this pose can help stimulate the organs in the abdomen, enhancing digestion and improving the functioning of the kidneys and bladder.

Promotes Pelvic and Lower Back Health: Regular practice of this pose can strengthen the muscles of the lower back and improve the stability of the pelvic region, which is beneficial for posture and overall back health.

Mental Benefits:

Reduces Stress and Anxiety: The seated, meditative nature of Butterfly Pose helps to calm the mind, reducing feelings of stress and anxiety.

Enhances Focus and Calm: As with many yoga poses, the focus on breath and posture during Butterfly Pose can improve mental clarity and focus.

Therapeutic Benefits:

Relieves Menstrual Discomfort and Menopause Symptoms: The opening of the hips and the gentle pressure on the abdomen can help alleviate discomfort associated with menstruation and menopause.

Beneficial for Prostate Health: The stimulation of the pelvic region is also beneficial for maintaining prostate health and can help alleviate symptoms of urinary disorders.

Additional Benefits:

Facilitates Childbirth: For pregnant women, practicing Butterfly Pose can help prepare the hips and pelvic muscles for childbirth, though it should be practiced with caution and possibly under supervision as the pregnancy progresses.

Improves Circulation in the Lower Body: The position of the legs and the gentle forward bend can help improve blood circulation in the lower body.

Caution:

While Butterfly Pose is generally safe, it should be practiced with care by those with knee or hip issues. Using cushions or blocks under the thighs can help reduce strain on these joints if the stretch feels too intense.

Overall, Butterfly Pose is a versatile and beneficial yoga pose that supports both physical and mental health, making it a valuable addition to many yoga practices.

Corpse Pose (Savasana)

Body Scan Meditation
Practice: Lie down or sit comfortably. Starting at your feet and moving up to your head, focus your attention on each part of your body in turn. Notice any sensations, tension, or discomfort without trying to change anything. Use your breath to release tension as you move through your body.
Benefits: Relaxes the body, reduces physical tension and stress, and improves body awareness.

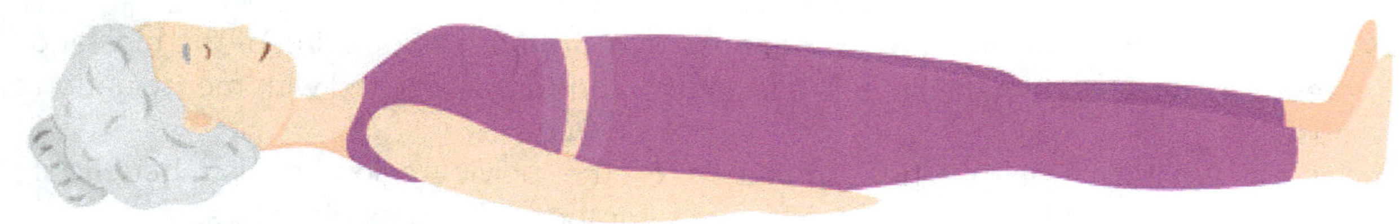

Conclusion

Congratulations on completing your journey through Yoga for Seniors or Beginners! Throughout this book, you've explored the transformative practices of yoga, meditation, and breathing techniques and delved into the fascinating world of chakras. Each page was designed to educate, inspire, and guide you toward excellent health, inner peace, and spiritual awareness.

As you close this chapter, remember that yoga practice is a continuous journey rather than a destination. The tools and insights you've gained are stepping stones to a more balanced and harmonious life. You can cultivate a sense of well-being through gentle postures, calming breaths, or deep meditative practices at any age or stage.

I encourage you to revisit these teachings often, integrate them into your daily routine, and continue to explore the depths of yoga and meditation. Each practice aims to deepen your understanding and connection to your body, mind, and spirit. Share your experiences with others, and may you continue to grow and thrive in your yoga practice.

Thank you for allowing us to be a part of your yoga journey. Namaste!

<u>Please share your experience and leave a positive review on Amazon.
It would warm my heart and help guide others to this same path of
discovery and wellness. Your words can light the way for someone searching for
a change, offering them the same hope and guidance you found in these pages.</u>

Copyright © By Mila Grace